Outsmarting
Managed
Care

Outsmarting Managed Care

A Doctor Shares His Insider's Secrets to Getting the Health Care You Want

Bruce A. Barron, M.D., Ph.D.

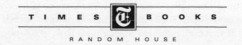
TIMES T BOOKS

RANDOM HOUSE

ISBN: 0-8129-2981-0

Random House website address: www.atrandom.com

Printed in the United States of America

98765432

First Edition

Book design by H. Roberts Design

SPECIAL SALES
Times Books are available at special discounts for bulk purchases for sales
promotions or premiums. Special editions, including personalized covers,
excerpts of existing books, and corporate imprints, can be created in large
quantities for special needs. For more information, write to Special Markets,
Times Books, 201 East 50th Street, New York, New York 10022, or call
800-800-3246.

This book is dedicated to all my patients
and to MCB for her patience.

ACKNOWLEDGMENTS

I am indebted to Pam Bernstein for her support and encouragement in undertaking this concept and selling it. Without the supervision, direction, and guidance of Betsy Rapoport, my editor at Times Books, this would have been a painful task rather than an educational experience, and by a country mile, it would have been an inferior book.

CONTENTS

Author's Note

I've written this book to help you work more effectively with your doctor and other health care professionals. This book is not intended to replace the role of your physician in diagnosing and treating illness. I have disguised the names and identifying characteristics of the patients described in this book to protect their privacy.

PREFACE

Your doctor has been serially morphed from a primary care physician into a health care provider and now is a gatekeeper. Dr. Jones has merged his practice with Med-Surg-Ped-Ob-Gyn-Psych Associates Inc. The office is now where a Blockbuster Video used to be in the mall.

Your medical insurance company was amalgamated with a larger company before being bought out by a new conglomerate with divisions that manufacture athletic equipment, fuel injection systems for small jet airplanes, and products made from recycled automobile tires. An initial public offering was made and it was transformed to a for-profit company, USA-Gibraltar-Cambridge Health and Healing Company.

It's Friday night. Your husband has had the sudden onset of crushing chest pain. Your five-year-old spikes a fever of 104. It's the eighth day of your period, you have begun to bleed very heavily and are passing large blood clots.

You're frightened and place a call to your doctor. On the twenty-third ring, the service answers. "Med-Surg-Ped-Ob-Gyn-Psych Associates Inc. Please hold."

After you have heard the complete collection of Elton John's Greatest Hits and half the score of Andrew Lloyd Weber's *Phantom of the Opera,* the line comes alive again. "Med-Surg-Ped-Ob-Gyn-Psych Associates Inc. Can I help?"

You tell the operator your problem.

"Dr. Friday is covering the practice. I will try to reach the doctor and have her call you back."

You have never met Dr. Friday and emphasize your concerns.

Taking your justifiable concerns as a personal affront, the operator says petulantly, "In that case, maybe you better go to the emergency room!"

"My insurance plan is the USA-Gibraltar-Cambridge Health and Healing Company."

"Oh well," she says, "in that case, you better call them before you do anything."

You realize that is clearly good advice. The emergency 1-800 number is on the back of your membership card.

"USA-Gibraltar-Cambridge Health and Healing Company. If you are calling from a touch tone phone, press one."

You follow the direction.

"Welcome to the USA-Gibraltar-Cambridge Health and Healing Company. Please listen carefully to the following menu of options. You may interrupt the speaker at any time to make your selection. If you would like to receive information about the new USA-Gibraltar-Cambridge Health and Healing Company programs, press one. If you have a question about your current monthly USA-Gibraltar-Cambridge Health and Healing Company statement, press two. If you have a question about a previous USA-Gibraltar-Cambridge Health and Healing Company statement, press three. If you would like to place an order from the current USA-Gibraltar-Cambridge Health and Healing Company herbal medicine catalog, press four. If you would like to place an order from the USA-Gibraltar-Cambridge Health and Healing Company athletic clothing and sneaker catalog, press five. If you would like an application for membership in the USA-Gibraltar-Cambridge Health and Healing Company Health Club near you, press six. If you have a question about an unpaid claim, press seven. If your physician has complained to you about an unpaid claim, press eight. If you are a member of the USA-Gibraltar-Cambridge Health and Healing Company and this is an emergency, press nine."

When you press nine, you are told, "Please enter your twenty-seven-digit member number followed by the pound sign."

"You have entered zero-one-four-three-nine-one-six-six-three-one-zero-four-eight-six-two-five-five-nine-two-one-eight-seven-six-four-three-two-two. If this is correct, press star zero."

By now in a controlled rage and sweating, having successfully completed that awesome task, you are now instructed, "Please enter the eleven-digit number of your case manager found in the lower right corner of your membership card."

After you have been told how important your call is to them eleven times and enough time has passed to convince you that you have been disconnected and must resist the attempt to start pressing the buttons on the phone at random, you are informed, "Terry, your case manager, is not available. At the tone, you may record your message. If you need to speak with someone immediately, press one to speak with another case manager. To return to the main menu, press the pound sign."

You press one.

"All case managers are currently busy. Calls are answered in the order in which they are received. Your call is very important to us. Please remain on the line and the next available case manager will answer your call."

After you have heard the last half of the score of *Les Mís* and been informed twenty-five times that your call is very important, you are told, "Your call is being transferred to a case manager."

"This is Cassandra. Can I help?"

I am sure that after such an exchange, if your husband has not succumbed to cardiac arrest, your child has not had a seizure, or you have not fainted from loss of blood, you are just a few short steps away from insanity. You know you need help, but you are rightly convinced that you are not likely to get it from Cassandra.

The help you need is in this book. It is a practical manual for understanding and dealing with today's health care system. It will permit you to wend your way through the obstacles that have been devised and implemented by the USA-Gibraltar-Cambridge Health and Healing Companies of the world. You will learn how to get to the decision makers and persuade them to do the right thing. You will learn why it is better to have an operation on Monday morning than Friday afternoon. You will learn the important questions to ask, and how and when to ask them. And you will learn the right answers.

I have spent the last thirty years not only in the medical care system but on the staff of one of its most prestigious citadels. I have been there during the salad days when the physician was king. My decisions were unquestioned and my orders executed without hesitation. But it was a system not without its faults. Then came the changes that resulted in *my* having to alter how I practiced medicine. I knew these modifications would not improve the care my patients would receive, but they were necessary to preserve my sanity.

For example, I found that I had to lie to a case manager in order to have an eighty-year-old woman with diabetes and heart disease admitted to the hospital on the day before surgery for her ovarian cancer. It was important to have a full pre-op day to collect important data on the patient's current medical condition before exposing her to the enormous risks of surgery.

I had to spend more and more time documenting everything I did, for if it was not recorded in painstaking detail, the system maintained that it hadn't been done. To justify receiving a fifty-dollar fee, I had to have a written record that included the patient's complaint; the history of the events that led to the office visit; a review of the patient's respiratory, cardiac, gastrointestinal, endocrine, neurologic, urologic, genital, musculoskeletal, and psychological systems; pertinent past history; family and social history. All this before I performed and recorded the results of a complete physical examination followed by a detailed discussion with the patient and a recorded summary of all this in addition to the plan of treatment. This lengthy written record replaced what I will admit were often inadequate, unreadable notes. However, with the increasing threat of malpractice suits and the need to transmit this information efficiently to the increasing number of professionals included in the care of patients, the form and character of the written medical record had substantially improved long before the imposition of all these regulations by governmental agencies and managed care organizations.

I have had the opportunity to see the medical care system from a variety of positions, including a short stint as a medical director for policy at Empire Blue Cross/Blue

Shield, a major medical insurance company. From a medical consumer's point of view, I was "the enemy." That experience allowed me to learn about the operation of the health care system from the insurer's point of view. As a senior medical director for policy, I had the opportunity to see how the medical care structure can be shaped and manipulated in a way that, for all practical purposes, is unrelated to the immediate goals of caring for the sick. The priorities of an insurance company, regardless of its apparent fiscal foundation, for-profit or not-for-profit, are inevitably focused on the bottom line. Every corporate decision is viewed in significant measure with this in mind. Until I was a member of such an organization, the dollar costs associated with the care of a patient never occurred to me, and were, in fact, never a part of my thinking. I did or ordered to be done what was, in my opinion, in the patient's best interest. I never made a treatment choice based on its cost or selected one method of management simply because it was cheaper than another. It is just such considerations that are the primary policy drivers for a medical insurance company.

There is a line in the play *Fiddler on the Roof* where the central character, Tevye, after explaining how he has had to bend in order to adjust, making many compromises with life, says, "but if I bend that far I will break." I can attest to the fact that, in very short order, practicing physicians who enter the insurance arena will feel that they have met their match. At Blue Cross/Blue Shield, I learned that the medical insurance company follows a very different drummer, and quickly saw that the corporate medical insurance world is way out of my weight class. In the final analysis, I viewed my personal surrender as a metaphor for the medical profession's abdication to the insurance industry. With this book, I'll share what I've learned from both sides of the battle over the quality of your health care.

There are good, better, and best approaches to the problems you face in this vitally important and rapidly changing arena. Here is a map to help you maximize the likelihood of your getting to the right provider, being given the right treatment, and getting the best result when you are forced to deal with today's health care system.

Outsmarting Managed Care

Introduction

I realized that this kind of book was needed when it became clear to me that, in the not too distant future, we would be referring to this time as the era of the devaluation of medical care and the dumbing down of medicine. My own experience led me to worry about who would take care of *me* when I need medical care. And if *I* had this concern, I was convinced other people did, too. I wrote this book with your needs in mind and expect it to play that role as you wend your way through the maze of the "New Era Medicine."

If you think I am exaggerating the magnitude of the problem, how would you characterize the following scenario? Medicine, like other professions, deals with such an obscure, extensive, complex body of information that no outside group can adequately or effectively monitor its functions. So society grants it the privilege of supervising itself. Individual members of the profession are certified by the state only after receiving approval by a credentialing body of the profession.

American doctors, the majority of whom are male, have high social status, make a great deal of money, and have the power that comes with both. When I finished my medical training and began my practice, it was a simpler time for patients and physicians. Medicine was a cottage industry. There were approximately 300,000 physicians in the United States. In the main, they practiced alone or in small groups. Medicine was a retail service business. Physicians knew their patients and their patients got to know them. The physician-patient relationship was a relatively simple interaction.

For those of you old enough to remember Marcus Welby, M.D., that was the way it was. You can probably recall the name of your pediatrician as quickly as the name of your best friend in high school. That medical care system and the notion of "my doctor" and all that implies—which most Americans enjoyed for more than four generations—has been transformed in concept as well as practice. This has happened, in large measure, as a direct result of super-specialization and the development of new technologies.

It was these changes that contributed to the increasing general unrest with the profession, patients finding their physicians less accessible, physicians unwilling to spend time with their patients, and a system that was increasingly entrepreneurial. Many physicians demonstrated unbridled avarice, arrogance, and paternalism. Since, in the aggregate, every one of these complaints is valid, the profession could no longer pretend to occupy the moral high ground.

Medicine became a very big business. Now there are more than 730,000 physicians in the country. With this enor-mous increase in their number, there has been a corre-sponding increase in the variability among them. Health care is now the largest single sector of the American economy and represents a trillion dollars of the gross domestic product. It became clear to economists, politicians, and chief financial officers of corporate America that if we were to be competitive in a world market economy, the cost of health care could no longer grow at the same exorbitant rate, or continue to devour as large a part of the gross national product. The force driving the changes in the medical care system and the medical profession was not a result of widespread dissatisfaction with the quality of care available but with the increasing cost of providing that care. It was the recognition that medical care was not responsive to market forces that resulted in the coalition of big business and government to contain medical care spending in America.

Managed care became the banner slogan for the mechanisms to reduce costs and to stop—or reverse—the rate of increase in the cost of the delivery of medical care. So, managed care is a euphemism for managing costs.

In business terms, it is relatively simple to achieve such a goal. One way to do this is to reduce the total number of units of health care that are delivered. A second option is to reduce the cost of each of those units of delivered medical care, and a third is to eliminate coverage or place restrictions on the use of selected costly units of care, such as organ transplantation or the treatment of infertility. Each of these strategies is now being used under the pseudonym of managed care. We are reducing the payments to those who provide services. We are limiting the services that are provided. And we are restricting the treatment choices and options of those who require care.

An even more fundamental change is taking place. In the past, the physician's primary responsibility was to do everything possible for the patient. Now, in certain managed care organizational structures, physicians are responsible for a population of patients and a corresponding budget.

The historical physician-patient relationship has become a tripartite interaction that now includes the payer—the insurance company or managed care organization. The system of physician compensation—capitation—and risk sharing—capitation plus bonus, in which doctors are given a spending budget per patient—provides a financial incentive for the physician not to hospitalize patients, not to order expensive tests or perform costly procedures. In such a payer-designed system new questions are being asked. How will we decide between patients competing for limited fixed resources? Can someone with a lower level of clinical training provide the care that is required for a given task; for instance, will an advanced practice nurse do as well as a physician? Does an expectant mother need an obstetrician or can a nurse-midwife do the job? Will a baby suffer if a nurse practitioner does the examination rather than a board-certified pediatrician? Is a psychiatrist any better than a psychologist for a patient who is depressed or anxious?

These questions highlight the current dumbing down of medicine. Physicians are now identified as health care providers, as are nurses, social workers, psychologists, physical therapists, occupational therapists, nurse's aides, dieticians, laboratory technicians, pharmacists, emergency medical technicians, and other members of the health care team. This new label is one expression of the leveling process that brings physicians down from their customary lofty position as captain of the team, commanding general of the health care troops. They are no longer sovereign rulers and must share the decision-making process with lesser trained providers.

During the past five years, as a result of the combined actions of employers, insurance carriers, and governmental agencies, the current cost and projected increases in the cost of medical care have been reduced. But because there has been a widespread patient backlash to the unpalatable radical changes to the medical care system, it has been decided to pretend that these changes have occurred as a result of a fictitious "consumer demand." Politicians and professors alike are now suggesting that it is the smarter, time-pressed consumers—those savvy beings who have, in the past, changed other industries—who have health care in their sights. It is they who are demanding more convenient services, more information about them, and more respect for their knowledge about these services.

Regina Herzlinger, a Harvard Business School professor, has written about the new generation of consumers who are "tremendously assertive, pragmatic, and manipulative," which she attributes to a combination of more education and less free time. These people are less deferential to doctors and more willing to do their own extensive research to get health-related information. "Even if *you* don't think (patients) are smarter, they think they're smarter. . . . We're in an age where we're all equals," Professor Herzlinger writes.

The adoption of a corporate model for the medical care system has led to the formation of a host of new complex organizations and relationships. Under the name of managed care, the once simple interaction between doctors and patients has been modified to include health maintenance organizations (HMO), preferred provider organizations (PPO), independent practice associations (IPA), point of service plans (POS), primary care physicians (PCP), utilization management units (UM), quality assurance committees (QA), precertification review companies (PR), physician hospital organizations (PHO), medical service organizations (MSO), and physician practice management companies (PPM).

The widely advertised demonizing view of a health care

system dedicated to the self-interests of doctors, hospitals, and insurance companies has led to changes that are being too aggressively marketed. "Outcomes of Care" has recently been presented as a rallying cry of this new system in an attempt to dignify their new and untested programmatic initiatives and justify their implementation. Managed care companies have recognized the enormous complexity and inherent difficulty of rigorously determining the effects of medical treatment, and in response have introduced the "clinical guideline" as a working standard for high-quality care. These guidelines, however, may or may not be directly correlated to good or desirable outcomes. In other words, managed care organizations are asking providers to follow guidelines that may not have any relationship to how well you'll do after treatment—and that's the only standard you really need to worry about. If these newly introduced techniques required the approval of any regulatory agency such as the FDA, their introduction might possibly be justified. Lacking such oversight, the effects of the literally hundreds of practice guidelines issued by the vast majority of managed care organizations need precise evaluation. I will admit that these guidelines may constrain the incompetent and minimally competent physician to follow some sensible rules. However, at this point, these methods can, at best, be expected to elevate the bottom to the average. The question remains as to their effects on good doctors. The best guess is that while in the long run they will elevate the bottom up, at the same time they will pull the top down.

No one would suggest that these recipes will foster excellence. If we lose sight of such "excellence" as the ultimate goal for our system of medical care and allow the cost considerations to become paramount, I have grave doubts that excellent physicians will remain the hallmark of medical care in the United States. Once lost or compromised, excellence is not easily rediscovered or re-created. To strive for excellence is a form of elitism, but elitism is not necessarily a pejorative. I am sure you want your doctor to be excellent! In fact, we all want our doctors to be the best!

It was not until I confronted the system head-on as a patient that I decided I would write this book. I had been in practice almost twenty-five years, and in that time I had never been really sick. A few years ago, when I noticed a small sore on my knee, I was convinced I had developed a small area of eczema or psoriasis. I took out my old dermatology textbook and found that this is a common site for psoriasis—and a not uncommon occurrence in a sixty-year-old male. Satisfied with my diagnosis, I treated it with a variety of topical steroid creams. Two months later it had not only failed to respond to the various medications I had used but it was clearly larger. So one afternoon I walked down the hall and asked one of my colleagues, a professor of dermatology, to take a look at it.

"Psoriasis! Leave it alone!"

My opinion was confirmed. I stopped using the medicines. One month later it was even larger, so I decided to get a third opinion. I called the office of a colleague who had been chief resident in dermatology when I was an intern in medicine. When I asked for an appointment, his secretary questioned me extensively about my medical insurance and advised me, "You need a referral note from your PCP." I was aghast. I needed a referral from my primary care physician! This was a new experience and I bristled at her tone and manner. I was sufficiently imperious that she gave me an appointment for that morning. The conversation ended with her reminding me that since I had not fulfilled my deductible for the year I would be expected to pay 20 percent of the $350 fee at the time of the visit. "We accept Mastercard and Visa. A personal check will be satisfactory, too."

I was kept waiting thirty minutes after filling out a two-page form with equal parts of my personal, medical, and financial history. I was not feeling very collegial when, after sitting in a tiny examining room for an additional ten minutes, my colleague walked in. I apologized for forcing my way into his already crowded office hours, and we bantered for a few minutes about the old days. I then pulled up the leg of my trousers and showed him the lesion. He looked at it for about thirty seconds. "Could be Bowen's, but I think it's a squamous cell."

These two diagnoses were very different from psoriasis; squamous cell cancer had the potential for significant problems, including metastasis and death. "Not psoriasis?" I asked hopefully.

"I doubt it. We need a biopsy."

"Fine. Let's do it."

"We'll set up an appointment for next week."

I knew this procedure would take no more than five minutes at most. "Look, Harry, I am now a little anxious about this. Can't you do it right now?" He had, after all, included cancer among the possible diagnoses.

"I'm really backed up. Running late."

I guess the expression on my face was sufficient, or maybe he recalled that I had referred more than a few patients to him, but he changed his approach.

"Okay."

The whole procedure took less than five minutes. It was 10:30 A.M. We both knew it was possible to process the biopsy specimen overnight and the pathologist could read the slide in the morning. It would not take a herculean effort to have an answer for me by noon the next day. So I was surprised when he said, "I'll give you a call when I get the report next week."

"Next week!"

"Yeah. They're really backed up in the lab. I'll call you."

I decided not to pursue this issue with him. He and his secretary had made it clear that they had extended themselves much further than they thought was warranted on the basis of our professional relationship.

When I got back to my own office, I called the dermatology pathology lab. I was speaking to a secretary.

"This is Dr. Barron. I've just had a biopsy done of a skin lesion and I'm quite concerned since the doctor suggested that it might be a cancer. I wonder if you could possibly put it through as a rush?" It was a request I had made hundreds of times for my patients. She was most accommodating.

"Yes, of course."

"Could you call me with the result?"

"Of course. I'll call you tomorrow as soon as it is signed out."

She did call the next morning. The dermatologist was wrong. The diagnosis was a basal cell epithelioma. Although it would have to be removed surgically, it was nothing ominous.

When I told my nonphysician friends this story, they all laughed. Their uniform response to my dissatisfaction with the care I had received was that I had no idea what they had to put up with whenever they had to deal with any doctor, every hospital, and the entire medical system. They all find the health care delivery system fragmented, depersonalized, obscure, and expensive.

After living through this experience, which as a patient I found unacceptable, I listened to them with a different ear, and I realized that in many situations patients require an ombudsman, a knowledgeable advocate with unambivalent allegiance to them. Or, lacking that, a road map to help them find their way along what is often a bewilderingly complex, impersonal, and frightening journey through what I have come to characterize as the medical maze. I decided to provide such a resource.

I am convinced that it is your doctor whom you want to manage the care you receive. This book will help you deal with the layers of bureaucracy and institutional complexities that have been insinuated between you and your physicians.

While there is worldwide agreement that the best medical care in the world is found in the United States, it is also possible to get very bad care. This book will help you recognize the difference and provide you with the tools you need to access the best. If you are enrolled in a managed care program, it will help you understand the steps you must take to manage that system. If you are going to be hospitalized, it will provide you with a guide to minimize the likelihood that you will be subjected to the kind of care we read about in newspapers, hear on the radio, or see on television—the stories of patients who had the wrong leg amputated, the wrong kidney removed, who received the wrong medication or were incorrectly diagnosed and made sicker or even died as a result of bad medical care. Regrettably, these events are neither fiction nor are they rare. The knowledge you need to improve your chances that these untoward things will not happen to you is in this book.

CHAPTER 1

The Payers

Understand the Adversary

The health care system in the United States, which has the potential to deliver the best medical care in the world, is being transformed by the invasion of managed care. It's a whole new ball game. If you are enrolled in a managed care organization, you may have to change doctors, go to a new hospital, change the medications you are taking, or be unable to get the treatment your doctor wants you to have.

If you don't want to do these things, and you want to get the right doctor, have the best treatment, and have it paid for by your managed care organization, you have a lot of work to do and may have a fight on your hands. In order to overcome your adversaries, you should have a good idea who they are, where they come from, how they work, and the rules of their game.

* * *

At the end of World War II, and for the next twenty years, the vast majority of Americans purchased medical insurance independently—or were insured through their place of employment—from one of the almost seventy regional not-for-profit Blue Cross/Blue Shield plans. Medical insurance was available to everyone who could pay for it and there were astonishingly few rules or restrictions. Patients were free to choose any physician. It was not a perfect system, but its flaws had little impact on either your doctors or your medical care. The for-profit commercial insurance carriers had not made any significant inroads into the health insurance business.

As the medical insurance industry became more sophisticated and accumulated health data for the population, for-profit health insurance companies began to pick and choose those for whom they would provide insurance coverage. They began to exclude from coverage those at high risk, limiting themselves to those at low risk for needing medical care, a practice commonly known as "cherry picking." This left the take-all-comers, not-for-profit Blue Cross/Blue Shield plans, insuring the more expensive of us, those more likely to need care. This resulted in growing differentials in the cost of medical insurance between the not-for-profit and the for-profit insurance carriers.

It was economic forces that led to the profound changes in the organization of the health care system and payment for medical care. At the beginning of this decade, more than 90 percent of Americans who had medical insurance as a benefit of their employment received close to full payment for the cost of medical services provided under the supervision of the physicians of *their* choice. Today, in order to have the cost of their medical care reimbursed, almost 90 percent of the population of this country must choose doctors and hospitals approved by the managed care organization who pays the bill.

Managed care is a fragmented, money-driven, free-enterprise system. It is a very big business. The trillion-dollar American health care system is larger than the budgets of most countries, provides employment to some 9 million people, and represents almost 15 percent of the gross national product.

For the consumer, operationally, managed care means that there is a third party intimately involved in the details and decisions about medical care. Managed care means limitations in your choice of a doctor. Managed care means that your physician's fees are discounted. Managed care means there are restrictions on coverage for necessary services. These organizations decide what they will and won't allow, and unilaterally determine which and how many treatments they will pay for.

Physicians who work for managed care organizations are told how many patients they must see during a set of office hours. The managed care plan will in many cases restrict the medications a physician can prescribe to an approved list that may not include some a physician would prefer in a given clinical situation. The medical management of certain conditions may be specified with so-called practice guidelines developed by the managed care organization. And if a physician deviates from these protocols, he or she may suffer criticism, censure, and/or a financial penalty.

When you were handed the managed care organization's provider directory, from which you were to select your physicians, you implicitly accepted the judgment of the human resources and financial officers of your employer, who made the decision to select that particular managed care company. You must understand that this critical decision, in most cases, was made without any significant input by physicians or anyone else with the knowledge and experience to ask the right questions about medical care before making such a choice.

> As a managed care enrollee, your first operating principle is: It is very likely that at some point I will have to deal with the bureaucracy of my managed care organization.

Why Did This Happen?

Before 1990, the vast majority of physicians and hospitals had free reign. They could provide services at will, at prices they set without any regulation. The record shows that many physicians and hospitals behaved like pigs. Physicians' fees grew at rates not seen in any other segment of the economy as they often charged extravagant sums for the services they provided. The historic ethic of not-for-profit hospitals disappeared. Hospital administrators began to be paid like corporate chief executive officers. Many negotiated contracts with lavish perks and golden parachutes. Health insurers paid the bills that were submitted essentially without question. As a result, the cost for traditional fee-for-service medical care was rising by as much as 20 percent a year. So the short answer to the question "why managed care" is that medical care began to cost too much.

Articles began to appear in *The Wall Street Journal*, business magazines, and daily newspapers attacking the system, claiming it was on the brink of chaos and demanding radical change. Surveys revealed that the median income of cardiologists was $300,000; orthopedic surgeons made even more. Aware of these large and growing numbers and the historic immunity of the health care system to conventional market forces, it was a logical candidate for the imposition of some external form of fiscal control.

Corporate America became concerned. When Lee Iacocca learned that the cost to produce a single Chrysler automobile included $1,200 for health care for the employees and their dependents and only $500 for the steel, he knew it would be impossible for him to compete in the world market unless he could reduce the number of dollars the company spent on health care. And what was true for Chrysler was true for General Electric and Motorola and Exxon and so on and so on and so on. Corporate America decided to reinvent the nation's health care system along lines that were familiar to them, and so we have had the corporatization of American medicine.

Since benefits managers in large American corporations have apparently assumed that all health care plans deliver a product of at least acceptable quality, price became the primary factor in selecting one plan over another. These decision makers knew that if you pay for a Mazda you are not going to be driving a Mercedes, and the directors of managed care plans admitted that they were not going to spend significant amounts of money on care that was by and large unmeasurable, so the central issue of the quality of the care provided wasn't even addressed. In fact, Paul Elwood and the other fathers of managed care, known collectively as the "Jackson Hole Group," having met at Elwood's Jackson Hole, Wyoming, residence, recently confessed, with notable and shocking absence of contrition, that quality was not a factor of central interest to them.

> As a managed care enrollee, your second operating principle is: I must remember that if I need care, it is no longer just between me and my doctor.

What Happened?

The health care delivery system in the United States is undergoing a revolution that is best characterized as a shift from fee-for-service to managed care medicine. Ten years ago, Allied Signal, a corporation with more than eighty thousand employees, was one of the first major companies to transfer employees into a managed care program. This began what became a sea change in the way employers provided or facilitated the purchase of health insurance by their employees. Managed care plans generally offered two options: the "no choice, minimal cost to the employee" option and the "some choices with greater costs" option.

The majority of Americans are now participants in managed care programs, with 77 percent of Americans and their dependents insured through their employers. In addition, thousands of Americans covered by Medicare have enrolled in managed care plans that reduce their financial exposure when they are ill. For physicians, this redesign of the system has resulted in large decreases in their income. Managed care organizations are hiring salaried physicians and reducing what they pay participating physicians for the services they provide to their enrollees.

There is now ample evidence that managed care organizations are cutting down on treatment and dedicating savings to their bottom line. While there may be a public relations problem for a physician who has to explain an income of a million dollars a year, that is a minor issue compared to the one-hundred-million-dollar income of the CEO of a managed care company. The polarizing effects of this use of their insurance premium dollars has resulted in many large employers deciding to bypass managed care organizations and contract directly with hospitals and doctors. This is just beginning to happen and may well change the mechanics of the process. However, this is not going to help you, for patients and physicians alike dealing directly with employers promises not to be much different from dealing with managed care organizations.

Managed care has changed the system from one that perhaps tempted physicians to do too much—by rewarding them with fee-for-service compensation—to a system of restraints and constraints that can encourage them to do too little. It should not escape your notice that all this was done with the implicit promise that the quality of care would not be compromised while the cost of delivering that care would be contained. In many managed care plans, there are significant financial incentives to the physician that can hardly be expected to improve the quality of care provided. For example, physician productivity is encouraged through a compensation system that rewards physicians more for seeing the last patient in a day than for the first. This has not escaped the notice of managed care physicians. In order to maintain their productivity and income, there has been an increase in doctors' use of nurse practitioners to maintain the required patient volume. One quarter of physicians have reported that they are no longer able to make clinical decisions that are in their patient's best interest without the possibility of reducing their own income.

While there is no doubt that the current managed care movement is making great strides in the marketplace, it has not been a rousing success in the court of public opinion. Patients have become aware of the pressures on their physicians. Sixty-one percent of managed care patients believe their physician has decreased the time spent with them. Fifty-one percent have perceived a lower quality of care by their doctor. A majority of Americans now think the government should be involved in developing regulations to protect managed care enrollees from being treated unfairly.

Specifically, questions have been raised concerning how much time these plans provide for inpatient care for women being treated for breast cancer or who are admitted for maternity care. Currently more than a thousand legislative initiatives and regulations to control health plans have been introduced in thirty-nine states and more than a hundred have been initiated in Congress. There is a variety of informed opinions about these matters, and it is not at all clear that any of these issues warrant legislation.

Managed care companies have been very aggressive in attributing to their employers any change that is perceived by its enrollees—referred to as customers. They claim that if the business is trying to make deep cuts in the health benefits of its employees, it will choose a very restrictive plan that limits the choice of providers, treatments, and hospitals.

Patients' concerns have been mirrored by physicians. Three quarters of physicians included in a survey in Connecticut felt that the nonphysician reviewers employed by managed care companies impede patient access to care. Doctors are infrequently consulted as a source of information about the quality of the care that is delivered. Physicians have been critical of the process measures managed care plans use to evaluate physician performance. For example, the managed care plans want to know if doctors screen their patients for high blood pressure, perform screening mammograms, take Pap smears, and the like. Doctors reject these as appropriate indices of the quality of the care they are providing. While these organizations admit tracking these measures, simply doing so is a long way from the desired or expected treatment of a specific disease once it is diagnosed—and that, after all, is the real measure of the quality of medical care.

The Institute of Medicine, the medical division of the

National Academy of Science, has defined quality as "the degree to which health services for individuals increase the likelihood of desired health outcomes and are consistent with current professional knowledge." How do you know whether the quality of your medical care is average, below or above average, or superior? You must understand that this is a very complex question for which there is no good answer. Simply put, physicians view quality in medical care as the application of accepted standards of care based on the findings of rigorous clinical investigations. Patients, in contrast, often define quality by whether their doctor has a caring attitude and how he or she communicates with them, or how long they are kept waiting to see the doctor, rather than on the accuracy of the advice offered and treatment provided. Managed care organizations value patient satisfaction and respond to what patients think. This is a business decision. When patients are satisfied, they are likely to stick with their managed care organization.

The broadly based lack of interest in the quality of medical care is demonstrated by the results of a survey of 384 large corporations. Ninety-seven percent considered cost when choosing a health plan, only 29 percent considered quality. This was justified because both purchasers and consumers were primarily concerned with cost. Very few purchasers have ever terminated a contract with a managed care organization because the quality of care provided was poor.

These are not minor factors, and they have resulted in a conflict between professionalism and profit, between commercial and professional traditions in this country. While both have made significant positive contributions to our economy, the changes being implemented by the managed care system are affecting the medical care you receive.

While medical insurance has historically been almost exclusively the province of not-for-profit companies, the proportion of members in for-profit managed care plans has exploded from 12 percent in 1980 to more than 60 percent in 1998. The managing of costs and the drive to gain a larger market share by these companies have transformed the business of medicine into a market-oriented system.

One hallmark of these programs is the assignment of financial risk to physicians with respect to the cost of the care they provide their patients. While income incentives remind doctors that resources are limited and may encourage them to look for the most cost-effective method of treatment, when a doctor's income is based in large part on financial incentives not to treat patients, an ethical conflict is embedded in the relationship. Paying a flat fee per patient per month to the doctor is known as capitation. Often a variety of incentives and bonuses are added to the pay package of doctors based on their fiscal performance. The physician is not a free agent in these systems—that is, the doctor cannot just order up a test or procedure without considering its cost and potential impact on his or her income. Managed care companies usually retain external monitors who are in control of pre-approval for and utilization of many medical interventions. It is clear for many, many patients that, at some point, there will be an inevitable conflict of interest between the managed care plan's profit motive and the patient's need for excellent medical care.

To attach some numbers to the process of capitation, a typical primary care physician might have a thousand patients on his rolls. His or her base pay of $7 per patient per month (no, that is not a typo) generates his $7,000 monthly pay. He or she can qualify for an additional 50 percent bonus ($3,500) if he or she holds down hospital admissions, emer-

gency room use, and referrals to specialists. If his or her patients use more than a threshold value of inpatient days, he
or she loses all of the potential bonus. To collect the full
bonus, hospital use must be less than an established minimal number. A similar set of numbers is attached to the use
of specialists. This model clearly puts the physician at financial risk. In fact, your physician's income may be maximized
by minimizing the care provided his or her patients.

These changes in the medical care system are being implemented on the same basis and using the same methods
that have been used in other industries that have been
reengineered in the last ten years, and it has led to many,
many problems.

It will take some time before the outcomes of decisions can be rigorously examined to determine whether
such practices as discharging women from the hospital
within twenty-four hours after having a baby are justified. If
no disadvantage can be demonstrated by such an abbrevi-
ated hospital stay, it is likely that patient dissatisfaction with
such early discharge will have to be dealt with in other ways.

Currently, managed care organizations claim that as
many as 80 percent of their members are satisfied with the
care they are receiving. It is striking that in marked contrast
to these claims, objective polls of managed care enrollees
who become patients reveal widespread dissatisfaction at
having a third party inserted between them and their physicians. If the question is framed carefully, in terms of member
dissatisfaction with managed care, there are large and meaningful differences between enrollees in managed care plans
who rate their health plan fair or poor and those still using
traditional indemnity insurance.

With all the changes in the medical care system, consumers are more likely to rely on the marketing abilities and

perceived reputation of a managed care company, since in most cases specific data on physicians is very difficult to obtain or unavailable (see Chapter 2). Evaluations of quality that have been conducted suggest that managed care has not had a negative effect on the quality of care of the average patient. But it is far too early to come to a definite conclusion, and this does not appear to be the case for patients with significant illnesses.

Under managed care structures, a significant portion of revenues are diverted for such corporate objectives as dividends, advertising, and executive salaries, thereby reducing the amount of money that can be spent on patient care. It is inevitable that there will be a general downgrading of medical personnel, substituting less qualified and less experienced individuals who will accept reduced compensation.

When polled, doctors are nearly unanimous in their concern that the increase in managed care has had a negative impact on their clinical independence. Three quarters of those included in a survey felt that the quality of care had been negatively affected by managed care. In a parallel survey of patients, more than 80 percent reported that their managed care plan agreed with their physician's management decisions. This impression stands in stark contrast to studies that demonstrated that the shift of patients with heart disease or diabetes from cardiologists and endocrinologists to primary care physicians resulted in a lower rate of the use of resources and associated lower costs while at the same time the incidence of complications among these patients increased significantly.

There is an inherent conflict between the drive to balance business performance as expected by stockholders with the quality and quantity of care delivered to managed care enrollees. Managed care companies have fundamentally different goals than businesses whose profits are tied to increasing services delivered or products made and sold. For the company, profitability is a function of physicians doing less and patients receiving less care. For the share-holders, when more care is given, the value of their stock declines.

> Your third operating principle as a managed care enrollee is: It's not personal, but the managed care organization has an agenda that may result in decisions and actions that may not be beneficial to me.

The managed care companies have almost universally claimed that the source of their profits would come through the elimination of overuse, fraud, and abuse in the medical care system. They have taken the position that their actions will have little or no impact on the quality or amount of care provided to their enrollees. No one knowledgeable about current practices would challenge the assertion that medicine is far from perfect. One quarter of hospital deaths may be preventable, and as many as one third of some hospital procedures may expose patients to risk without improving their health. One third of drugs prescribed may not be indicated, and one third of laboratory tests showing abnormal results may not be followed up by the physicians who order them. Even more to the point, we know that the outcome of a procedure performed under perfect conditions is not an appropriate measure of the outcome of that same procedure under usual or average circumstances. The complication rates of many, many procedures performed by community-based surgeons are not as low and the outcomes not as good as among those in major academic medical centers. However, even with all these wasteful processes corrected, it is highly unlikely that the savings would equal the profits envisioned by the investors in for-profit managed care organizations.

In fact, many of the practices of managed care organizations appear almost to be *designed* to compromise the quality of care—and end up increasing the costs of delivering care. A case in point: Forty-seven-year-old John McCarthy began to experience chest pain. His primary care provider ordered a workup that didn't reveal the cause of his complaints. Under the assumption that his symptoms were a function of a gastrointestinal problem, she treated him with antacids and tried to persuade him to stop smoking and drinking his habitual six to ten cups of coffee each day. After a few months, he continued to complain of intermittent pains and underwent a second stress test. This time the results pointed to a problem with his heart, and after some discussion it was decided that he would undergo cardiac angiography to evaluate the status of his coronary arteries. At this point, it was the patient's understanding that if anything was found that should and could be corrected, it would be done at that time. After undergoing this invasive procedure with all its attendant risks, he was very upset to learn that although a blockage had been identified, nothing had been done, and he would have to return in ten days for the doctor to attempt to open the blocked artery in his heart through an angioplasty. Regrettably, he suffered a heart attack during the procedure, a known potential complication of angioplasty. The issue here is not the heart attack, but rather why the patient had to have two procedures in the first place. While it may sound harsh, the question must be asked: Did the fact that the managed care company would pay two separate fees, one for the initial angiogram and a second for an angioplasty, play any role in the physician's decision not to do everything at one sitting? There is an accumulating body of data that shows physicians are making decisions that are, in part, a function of the payment policies of the managed care organization. And often these decisions are not in the best interests of the patient.

An additional issue of the managed care organization's processes for controlling access to care involves the way a patient is referred for specialist care. In order for a primary care physician in a managed care organization to be a knowledgeable adviser with respect to any recommendation for a procedure, he or she must have information about the complication rate and experience of the surgeon to whom the patient is being referred. *None of this data is in the hands of the managed care companies.* Absent this information, you are being directed through unknown terrain by someone without a compass. New, very preliminary initiatives are under way to collect the data that would allow primary care physicians to compare the results of different specialists. At this time, however, there are no such resources other than the available databases described in Chapter 2.

In large measure, managed care organizations recruit physicians based simply on geography and their area of specialization. Under the managed care model, every patient has a generalist physician, commonly referred to as a primary care physician, or PCP, who provides both care and referrals to specialists. In order to be attractive to the largest number of people, managed care organizations want to maximize the number of generalist physicians participating in their plan. In fact, most managed care organizations actively recruit any generalist physician—including family practitioners, internists, pediatricians, and obstetrician-gynecologists—who passes their essentially uncritical screening procedures.

When you first enroll in a managed care program, you may find that your generalist primary care physician is not a participating provider. As a rule, it is usually not a problem for him or her to become one. However, to become a provider, your physician must be willing to go through the credentialing process. Other than the cumbersome process of completing what is often a complex application, you should be aware that there can be significant issues. Your physician may not want to become a participating provider in a specific managed care organization. If your physician is a member of a group, the managed care organization may require that the majority or all the members in the group join the managed care program as well. The fee schedule may not be acceptable to your physician or his or her associates. Your physician may find it unacceptable that he or she be required to see you and receive a fee that is 25 or even 50 percent less than his or her standard fee for an office visit. In addition, there are usually specific enrollment periods for physicians that may be limited to one or two months a year.

A different agenda is involved in the enrollment of specialist physicians—surgeons, urologists, orthopedists, and the like—in managed care plans. For financial reasons, it is in the interest of the managed care organization to limit the number of participating specialists and approved hospitals participating in their programs. In this way, they can ensure that they control a meaningful portion of the patient load of a given specialist or hospital. This has proven to be a successful business strategy in terms of having the upper hand when negotiating specialist fees and hospital charges. Again, there has been no uniform effort to develop methods that would permit the rigorous evaluation of the quality of care that is provided to their enrollees other than collecting on-going data on malpractice suits and negative actions taken by a hospital where the physician has admitting privileges. And there are some political forces that have proposed that managed care companies be required to include in their network any willing provider with the appropriate state medical license.

While it has been shown that the observed large differences in survival among patients who have heart attacks is a function of where they are hospitalized and who takes care of them, the fact is that the procedures and practices of managed care companies limit the referral options of primary care physicians. The data for heart attack victims is similar for patients with other significant illness: Where one receives care can be the single most important determinant of the quality of care that is provided. Your physician's hands may be tied even when he or she is aware of differences in survival data for the hospital to which you are being referred.

> As a managed care enrollee, your fourth operating principle is: I must make the effort to understand the qualifications and limitations of the participating providers and hospitals.

There are many situations where no provider in a managed care network is among the best for the treatment of a specific condition. It may also be true that the best hospital for the treatment of your condition is not a participating institution in your managed care organization. Under these circumstances you are going to want to go "out-of-network" for care. Unless the problem is one that the managed care organization has "carved out" so that patients are automatically referred to nonparticipating providers and hospitals, this will involve your entering into what you will in all likelihood become an adversarial process with your managed care company (see p. 48).

(see p. 48)

* * *

A reduction in the development of new medical technologies is another reasonable expectation from the expansion of managed care programs. While there has been a doubling of the number of physicians per capita and a tripling of health care spending as a percent of the nation's gross domestic product from 1960 to 1995, during this same period there was an eightfold increase in the cost of medical care directly attributable to technological advances. There is no doubt that the pace of discovery and the implementation of these innovations will decline because of the reduction of the funds allocated to the medical care system. In fact, it has already been shown that expenditures are down among Medicare beneficiaries who live in areas where managed care has made a high penetration. They have received fewer or less intensive services than Medicare beneficiaries in areas where managed care has not yet established a significant presence.

To get an idea of the magnitude of the effects of medical technologic advances on the cost of care, consider the cost of new surgical procedures on the brains of patients with Parkinson's disease; or the new drugs for the treatment of multiple sclerosis, which can cost $12,000 a year and surpass in effectiveness the pills currently prescribed that cost a few cents a day; or the tripling in price for improved inhalers for patients with asthma. If you multiply these increases in costs by the more than one hundred significant new and better therapies introduced every year, you can appreciate the increase in the cost of delivering medical care due to these advances.

Why It Won't Work

Like any other service or commodity, the health care system is dependent upon money. At first glance, it looks like any other market entity. It has a revenue stream derived from sales of services and products. It has expenses—the cost of personnel and supplies, and the creation and maintenance of hospitals. Managed care organizations can be as large as Columbia-HCA or as small as a single doctor's office. These organizations can be for-profit or not-for-profit. They can be nongovernmental or agencies of a government. Until 1970, the health care system operated in a relatively unfettered and unregulated environment. It was and still is viewed by many like any other market commodity.

The fact that has been overlooked is that health care does not act and cannot be perceived to behave like a normal market. Americans as a group view health care as an essential human service. Some consider it an essential right. The public unanimously believes that they should have access to all the medical care they need and that it should be of the highest quality. This stands in stark contrast and is not consistent with a structure that is subject to conventional market forces.

There is an almost universal concern about the appropriate role of money in health care. Patients usually find it difficult to talk about how much their care will cost lest they appear to be more concerned about their money than their health. It is astonishing how infrequently they ask about physicians' fees. Physicians as a group are equally uncomfortable talking about what they charge for their services. They often escape this task by delegating any such discussions to a member of their office staff. These behaviors are not replicated in any other area of our economy.

Investment bankers have found health care to be fertile ground. The public has been outraged by the millions that have been paid to executives in health care management companies whose salaries and bonuses have reached the stratospheric heights of such superstars as Michael Jordan or Barbra Streisand. The enormous sums involved in this business have been highlighted by the series of scandals that have gone beyond civil offenses of fraud and abuse of the system and now, in a few instances, include alleged criminal activities that look amazingly like racketeering.

The money that is being made by these investor-owned organizations, now the middlemen in the process, was formerly paid to physicians, other health care providers, and hospitals. In the change to managed care, we have lost sight of the goal of allocating the largest number of health care dollars to patient care and public service. In a free enterprise, entrepreneurial system, it is inevitable that some will enter the health care field primarily for money. But if, as it appears is happening, under our new operating models of the health care system, we lose sight of the social context of health care as manifest by the public's perceptions and patients' expectations, there will be increasing dissatisfaction and distrust, which will lead to an even louder call for government action to protect those at risk in the system: you.

There are some who believe that the managed care movement is going to fall of its own weight. They have come to this conclusion for a variety of reasons based on some variation of the assumption that consumers of medical care value a relationship with a physician above any other in the delivery system. While it is difficult to take issue with this premise, since historically physicians have played the pivotal role in directing their patients, more recently patients have come to view their relationship with providers as one that requires continuing critical examination and vigilance.

It has become obvious, as the managed care companies have started to increase the premiums paid by their enrollees, that there are significant problems with the system. They have concentrated their efforts on managing costs. They have reduced the length of hospital stays and at-

tempted to implement changes to deliver care more sys-
tematically. But their primary focus has been market share,
and this has led to a bidding war for customers that artifi-
cially lowered premium costs. Doctors and hospitals have
been forced to accept lower rates of reimbursement for the
services they provide. Now all these short-term measures
have run their course, and the real costs of managed care
programs are emerging.

The providers—individual physicians, group practices,
hospitals, and health care systems—have recently acknowledged that they have had to offer improved service of a
demonstrably high quality at a low cost. Their very expensive marketing and advertising programs are being developed to emphasize these strengths in order to maintain and
expand their core business, outpatient and inpatient care.

The fascinating part of this exercise is that it is the
providers—the doctors and hospitals—who possess the basic
data that is of any use in this process. The managed care
companies do not have this information. The only clinical
data they have comes from their panel of providers. The
doctors and hospitals are beginning to recognize this advantage and are flexing their considerable collective muscle
to organize, analyze, and present their findings to the marketplace. As this inevitably becomes a widespread practice,
the health plans will be forced to enter into cooperative ven-
tures with the providers on a far more equitable basis than
is currently the routine practice.

It is likely that the increasing organization of primary
care physicians will also dilute the influence and power of
the managed care companies. The development of single
and multispecialty groups of providers will also diminish
the ability of the managed care organization to control the
vital elements of its own balance sheet. The recent flood of
consolidations and mergers of hospitals, creating larger and

larger health care delivery systems caring for increasing numbers of patients, has enhanced their ability to facilitate the creation of dedicated physician groups and has placed them in a position to bring the managed care companies to the bargaining table, where the negotiations are between equals.

As this process evolves, it will become evident that managed care companies are neither designed nor equipped to provide either management or care. It is now becoming clear that it is the providers who are best suited for this role. For these reasons, the managed care organizations are in the active stage of evolving. It is neither obvious nor easy to predict what their final form will be.

Alternative Forms of Managed Care Organizations

Health Maintenance Organizations

A health maintenance organization (HMO) is a managed care organization that is composed of a broad-based group of providers brought together by an insurance carrier. It is the least expensive form of managed care organization with the lowest premiums and the most restrictive practices. It is a prime example of the principle that you get what you pay for. If you choose to enroll in an HMO, you must choose a primary care physician (PCP) from among the panel of physicians included in that group. The PCP will act as your personal health care consultant, will coordinate your care, and is the resource who will decide when and to whom you should be referred for specialty care. A network of specialist physicians has also been established by the insurer. All fees for outpatient and in-hospital care supplied by network doctors and approved facilities are paid in full by the plan. With the exception of any carve-outs for particular problems, there are no out-of-network benefits available in an HMO plan.

The structure of an HMO permits the delivery of medical care for a relatively low cost because the providers in the panel have agreed to negotiated reduced rates of payment for their services, and in some instances have accepted a fixed payment for all the services they provide to patients enrolled in their panel. This method of payment has come to be known as risk-sharing. As I've mentioned, for the physicians in the panel there is a financial *disincentive* for them to provide extensive or expensive services. As a result of these payment structures, certain patients were not told of all the options for care, since it was against the financial self-interest of the HMO. Such practices have led to the passage of government regulations prohibiting HMO's from "gagging" their physicians—that is, preventing them from telling patients about appropriate albeit expensive treatment options. There is, however, no surefire way to know if your physician has been "gagged."

Point of Service Programs

Point of service (POS) programs involve higher costs but allow more flexibility in terms of provider choice. The subscriber will select a PCP who will play the same gatekeeper role as for the HMO subscriber, and referrals are required for care provided within the network. An out-of-network option can be used that is associated with higher deductibles and copayments paid by the subscriber.

Preferred Provider Organization

A preferred provider organization (PPO) is another form of managed care organization program. It is less restrictive than a POS program and involves higher out-of-pocket costs and a higher premium. A copayment for a portion of professional service fees and medications used is commonly a part of the PPO program. The PPO permits the subscriber to utilize in-network benefits without prior referral by the primary care physician. Out-of-network care is available where the subscriber pays for any charges above the managed care organization's schedule of fees for services rendered.

The fifth operating principle for you as an enrollee in a managed care organization is: There are exceptions to every rule.

Managed Care Organizations: How They Work

The fundamental changes in medical care for patients enrolled in a managed care organization involves some level of restriction of their choice of physicians, treatments, and place of treatment. The control of the managed care program's network of participating providers and institutions is in the hands of what have come to be known as utilization or case managers.

These medical decision makers are most usually nurses who can refer problems to physicians but in the main make decisions that patients have historically expected physicians to make. The rules governing utilization management in managed care organizations have taken this crucial role out of the hands of physicians and placed it with administrators whose overriding concern is saving the company money. With very, very few notable exceptions, these are for-profit organizations that rigidly control costs. It is as a result of their number-one priority that you may not get the most appropriate treatment.

Managed care companies have been shown to deny claims by asserting that required services are "not medically necessary," "not proven effective," or "experimental." While in some cases the patient has gotten the necessary care and the doctor has not been paid, more frequently the utilization manager has denied the care that was recommended by a physician and the patient didn't get the treatment.

Evaluating Health Care Plans

Before selecting any one medical plan, you should evaluate the level of coverage and costs associated for each of the following services:

- Primary care office visits
- Specialist office visits
- X-ray and laboratory services
- Immunizations
- Well-baby care
- Prenatal maternity care
- Outpatient services, including diagnostic testing and therapeutic procedures
- Hospitalization
- Emergency room visits
- Nursing facility charges
- Mental health care, inpatient and outpatient charges
- Care for substance abuse
- Prescription drugs with any limitations or exclusions
- Surgery, including anesthesia services
- Speech therapy
- Occupational therapy
- Physical therapy
- Rehabilitation services
- Home health care

- Hospice care
- Costs for ambulance services
- Provision for medical care when traveling outside the region of the network
- Private duty nursing
- Provision for the cost of highly specialized services such as in-vitro fertilization
- Elective procedures such as sterilization procedures and voluntary abortions

The National Committee for Quality Assurance (NCQA) has been designated by the managed care plans themselves as its appropriate rating agency. NCQA accreditation involves a survey of the plan that focuses on credentialing of physicians, the policy of informing members of their rights and obligations, available preventive health services, utilization management practices, record-keeping, and follow-up. It is up to the plan as to whether or not it wants to participate in such a review. Currently, fewer than 25 percent of all HMOs in the country have been fully accredited by the NCQA.

These reviews do make an oblique attempt to measure performance. As the executive vice president of NCQA has put it, "To evaluate a student who has been assigned homework, you could ask: Did he take his work home with him? Did he work at it for two hours? Did he turn it in on time?" These are important questions and may give you some lead as to how that student will perform, but what really matters is: Did the student get the answers right? Fundamentally, that is what is important to the patient. NCQA has developed an instrument to take such measures of a managed care plan's activities: the Health Plan Employer Data and Information Set (HEDIS). The variables in HEDIS measures include whether or not children are given immunizations at the right time or women have Pap smears and mammograms regularly. Such things are easy to measure. The much more important questions are: If the patient has breast or cervix cancer, was it detected or was it missed? The NCQA is now revising HEDIS measures in an attempt to get some answers to this type of question. By their own admission, they have a very long way to go.

The NCQA has issued a report that revealed widespread variation among the managed care organizations, or MCOs, in the country on nine separate measures ranging from early care for expectant mothers to the treatment of patients who have suffered heart attacks. The difference between the best and the worst of plans represented thousands of patients who received less than optimal and at times unacceptably low quality of care by NCQA's standards. But it appears that patients in the average plan may have received as good or better care than patients covered by traditional fee-for-service indemnity insurers.

An even more comprehensive report on the quality of managed care programs found that only 61.9 percent of patients who had suffered a heart attack had been treated with the drugs that would reduce the risk of a subsequent heart attack and death. The performance by plan ranged from as low as 10 to a high of 100 percent. The astonishingly wide variation in this measure of quality is a reflection of physician competence, and not of the plan itself. The huge variation in care in MCO programs is further documented by the finding that, in New England, 81 percent of children under the age of two receive appropriate immunizations, while only 59 percent of those in the Rocky Mountain states do. There were other variations within regions of the same order of magnitude.

Although the available data provide glaring evidence of the unacceptably large variance with regard to the quality of medical care that HMO members receive, this same report found that 56 percent of those enrolled in managed care programs were either "completely" or "very" satisfied with their current health plan. This discrepancy is a reflection of the inability of patients to evaluate the quality of the care they are receiving under their managed care program.

The NCQA is now undertaking a major overhaul of its accreditation process. Their measures of care are based on the use of preventive strategies and screening for undiagnosed disease, and not on the outcome of treatment of sick patients. The NCQA is now attempting to develop instruments that will allow the measurement of treatment results.

The NCQA had announced that, beginning in 1999, they would include in the accreditation process for health plans performance measures of care provided to their enrollees. Instead of plans merely being accredited, provisionally accredited, or denied, plans will be classified as excellent, commendable, acceptable, or denied. Recently, the implementation date for this program was put off to 2000. An excellent plan would deliver the highest quality of care and service with the medical management systems far exceeding the NCQA requirements. Less than 10 percent of plans are expected to be rated as excellent. A commendable plan delivers high-quality care and service that exceeds the NCQA requirements. An accredited plans delivers care and services that meet the NCQA standards. A provisional plan is in partial compliance with the standards with no deviations from those requirements that would be judged to pose a significant risk to the quality of care. A plan is denied if it has serious flaws in its systems. To find out your MCO's current NCQA rating, contact the chief medical officer of the managed care organization.

U.S. News & World Report has also become involved in evaluating managed care plans, publishing the results of their review. In their most recent survey (1998), they concluded that there was no easy way to tell which managed care organizations could be counted on to be consistently better than others. They candidly predicted that consumers are likely to be confused and frustrated in their attempt to make an educated choice of a managed care plan for many years to come.

In their recent review, the magazine presented a numerical ranking of 223 health maintenance organizations in forty-six states. The plans were ranked on seventeen measures that the magazine suggests are related to the quality of care provided. Yet none of the indices they included is a measure of the outcome of care a plan has provided to its enrollees. In other words, not one of the measures indicates how well patients actually do. This is a major flaw that compromises the utility of this effort.

While managed care companies themselves continually survey their enrollees to gauge "patient satisfaction," no one seems to have a clear understanding of how to design these subjective surveys, let alone interpret the results. There are no rigorous standards. The AMA has one view, the American College of Physicians another, and each health plan has its own survey and methodology for reporting their findings. A review of a number of these polls reveals that consumers don't seem to pay a lot of attention to quality measures. They assume that they are going to get good medical care. In the face of what really happens—in terms of the quality of medical care—this is a fundamentally flawed assumption. Patients make it clear in their survey responses that service is most important to them as demonstrated by how long they have to wait for an appointment, how they feel after having been seen by their doctor, and if they can see the person they want. These subjective measures have absolutely nothing to do with the ability or skills of their physician or the likelihood that they will receive good medical care.

A review of these surveys reveals that communication is the single most important index in patient's judgments about a doctor. Communication style drives all measures of patient satisfaction. If patients are happy about the doctor's overall style, they will put up with substantial inconvenience and overlook or ignore—and, astonishingly, forgive—marginal medical care.

Regardless of these recognized limitations, managed care companies have put great stock in these surveys. They spend a great deal of money in conducting them and give their participating physicians a report card based on the results. These report cards are not unimportant. If the payer gets numerous complaints about a doctor, it will be brought to his or her attention. If the physician refuses to accept this criticism, he or she could be removed from the registry of participating providers. More commonly, companies urge the doctor to fix the problem by the time of the next report card. If the problem isn't fixed, the doctor will generally incur some penalty. This can include a reduction in the rate of reimbursement as well as termination of the physician's contract with the managed care company. Whatever the outcome, customer satisfaction has now become as important an index in the health care business as it is for McDonald's, Sears, Ford, and General Electric. Physicians have been warned: Learn to pay attention to your customer's complaints. You either fix the problem or find another line of business.

Some physicians have admitted that these surveys have resulted in their modifying their own behavior with patients. One doctor faced with criticism about long waiting times instructed his secretary to add the names of fictitious patient emergencies into each list of office hours so as to have a ready explanation for being late.

Managed Care—The Doctor's View

For the practicing physician, perhaps nothing has changed the patient-physician interaction more than the advent of managed care. While it is true that, nationally, more than 92 percent of physicians have contracted with at least one managed care company, this has been an almost universally unwelcome change. Many, many doctors are now very unhappy with the quality of their professional lives.

The litany of physicians' complaints includes frustrations in their ability to deliver first-rate care, limitations on their control over their own office hours, financial incentives that compete with their professional obligations, and loss of autonomy and control over clinical decisions. It is clear that a new set of stresses has been superimposed on the ones that have historically been associated with the practice of medicine.

While there is some debate about the extent of physician disenchantment and defection, there is no question that there is strong evidence that ultimately this combination of responses will have a significant negative effect on the level of excellence of medical care that is available here. As the editor of the *New England Journal of Medicine* has declared, "One thing we know: disgruntled, cranky doctors are not likely to provide outstanding medical care. Payers, insurers, and legislators must recognize this predicament and stop pretending that doctor discontent doesn't matter." I would suggest that it is the patients for whom this epidemic of professional discontent is most important.

From the first day I went into practice, I asked each patient at her first visit, "How did you get to me?" The answer was invariably "My doctor, Dr. Smith, referred me to you," or "I called the referral service at the medical center," or "A patient of yours, my friend, Mrs. Jones, told me about you."

Patients came to my office with a mind-set that made this introductory visit comfortable for them and easy for me. They had information that resulted in a naturally positive bias. They had heard I was a "good doctor." They wanted to like me. They believed I would take good care of them. The tone and flavor of these first visits and our subsequent relationship was in large measure established as a result of their preconceptions.

The first visit with patients who were enrolled in a managed care program could not have been more different. The response to my opening question was simply "You are on the list." As a group, these individuals have been presented with a book that lists their program's participating doctors by specialty. Usually, within each field, an alphabetized list is presented by geographic region. In most cases, patients made it perfectly clear that I was chosen because my office location was convenient. This can hardly be viewed as likely to support, let alone enhance, one's self-esteem. I am convinced that it is also true that many found themselves in my office because my last name begins with a B and not S—or worse, Z.

For the managed care patient, the relationship with a doctor begins and continues on an entirely different basis. In many cases, there is a quite natural suspicion. In not a few cases, I have had to deal with patients' anger and hostility at finding themselves most reluctantly in a strange doctor's office because "My doctor is not in the plan my employer signed up with." It took some time for me to rationalize this adverse response and understand that, in many cases, these people were responding to the many horror stories about managed care that have appeared in the media.

It cannot escape any physician's notice that patients enrolled in managed care programs are highly focused on the cost of care. A recent study found that 26 percent of health plan enrollees switch to a cheaper plan when the monthly premium for their own plan increases by as little as ten dollars a month. This happens regardless of the fact that such a change will result in their having to change their physicians. This dominance of the cost factor creates a discrepancy between the theory of the importance, imputed value, and specificity of the patient-doctor relationship and the current practices of the patient in the health care system. Since employees are so sensitive to price differences, physicians have come to the reluctant acceptance that their relationships with patients enrolled in managed care programs are at best fragile and easily disrupted. For physicians, it takes a lot of accommodation to accept that this is not personal. I am still doing battle with the concept that regardless of what I do, my managed care patients have no firm allegiance to me. I have had to accept that profoundly unpleasant change in the tone and flavor of the relationships in my professional life.

In addition to these issues, I must admit that I am also struck by the marked decrease in my compensation for caring for managed care patients. Physicians who have agreed to participate in a managed care program have voluntarily agreed to discount their fees. These rate reductions range from 25 to 50 percent and occasionally more. The patients are expected to pay the five-, ten-, or rarely fifteen-dollar co-pay that is their responsibility according to their managed care plan. This means that they will pay an amount, out-of-pocket, that is less than the cost of two movie tickets or lunch at McDonald's. In financial terms, for both the patient and the physician, this has become an undervalued interaction.

The pay for doctors has leveled out. Between 1993 and 1995, the inflation-adjusted pay of most high-tech medical specialists fell from 3 to 10 percent. While their average incomes were still comfortably in the six figures, the chance of earning stratospheric incomes has dwindled. This has happened as a result of managed care.

Because patients switch doctors and insurance plans as often as they change jobs, managed care companies place small value on a single physician's practice, and indeed recognize not much more in a small group practice. This is demonstrated by the very small sums paid to physicians who are working under a capitated rate that can be as little as $7 per patient per month. For $84, a physician is expected to provide primary care to a patient for a year. While younger physicians are not distressed by these changes, older physicians are leaving practices or relocating to areas in the country where managed care has not made significant inroads.

> The sixth operating principle that comes into play when you are a managed care patient is: Don't be confused; the people at the MCO are not your friends. They're not necessarily even on your side.

Managed Care Administrative Personnel

The really scary folks in the managed care business are the medical directors and case managers. The medical directors of these organizations have the authority to tell participating doctors what they can and cannot do. Most managed care programs have more than one medical director, and they have widely varying credentials. Some are in these positions because they didn't want to deal with the demands of clinical practice. Others have taken these jobs because they saw their incomes shrink as managed care made greater inroads into the patient base of their own practices. A few have been motivated by a messianic drive to affect the medical care of hundreds of thousands or even millions through this administrative venue.

For the patient, there are no uniform standards for medical directors, and certainly no uniformity in their decisions. Their mandate includes providing members with a wide choice of physician providers and ensuring that complete and accurate patient records are maintained and that physicians practice according to established quality standards. In any given case, if a physician deviates from the organization's standards, the medical director has the right to initiate disciplinary procedures that can result in the doctor being removed from the plan's roster of physician providers.

The medical director's primary responsibility, however, is to keep a tight rein on medical expenses, and this is accomplished through case managers. The case manager is the operational, front-line intermediary between the patient who requires care and the insurer who is paying the bill. While some insurers maintain their own team of case managers, others have contracted with other organizations to which they have delegated this responsibility.

There is no accurate count of the total number of case managers presently in business, but eighteen thousand have been certified by the Commission for Case Management Certification, which was created in 1993. While many case managers are nurses, many are not. Regardless of their training, when case managers are confronted with a problem with which they have no experience, they are usually able to consult a medical director for advice. Regrettably, in many cases this is of little help, since both may have limited or no experience with a given problem and may not understand all the potential benefits or risks of a specific treatment plan. As a group, they often respond to problems based solely on cost considerations. But as has been pointed out, all decisions made by case managers and medical directors alike are subject to negotiation.

Doing Battle with Your MCO

The fundamental change in medical care for patients enrolled in a managed care program is the imposition of some restrictions in their choice of physicians, treatments, and place of treatment. Each program establishes a network of what are termed participating providers and institutions and a structure known as utilization management. While in many cases these limits may not be onerous, there is an increasingly large body of data to demonstrate that if you have a significant illness, the policies of the managed care organization may lead to restrictions that substantially increase your risks of an adverse outcome, including significant morbidity and mortality.

This point has been made most convincingly in two different studies of the problems encountered by diabetic patients and patients with heart disease whose cases were supervised by primary care physicians as contrasted with a group who were managed by physicians who had specialty training and qualifications.

The press has already reported the furor that arose with regard to the restrictions in the length of the in-hospital stay for women following an obstetrical delivery, and more recently attention has been paid to what was called the "drive-through mastectomy." It is not surprising that the American Association of Health Plans (AAHP), the umbrella group that represents managed care plans, has mounted many public relations campaigns to explain away the limitations of access to care by members of managed care plans, the incentives to physicians and other health care providers to undertreat, and the glaring loss of physician's autonomy. They have now adopted a new initiative with the slogan "Putting Patients First." Their current promotional campaign is very sketchy with regard to operational details, but they are aggressively accusing the media of making an issue of the supposed unsavory practices of managed care companies where none exist. AAHP recently admitted that it urged its members not to push women undergoing breast cancer surgery out of the hospital too soon. There is evidence that this policy statement was made, in part, to stave off legislative initiatives. Overall, this organization claims that Americans are in general satisfied with their health care coverage.

As it is unethical to do unnecessary procedures where fee-for-service rewards the physician with a financial gain, it is equally unacceptable for a physician to limit medical care to a patient under managed care for financial gain. It is clear that as a nation we are embarked on a path of health care reform that will result in cost control through managed care. This, it appears, will be achieved with the participation of promoters, marketers, lawyers, accountants, consultants, reviewers, and shareholders, all of whom share in the revenue stream before physicians are paid their portion of the health care premium.

This issue has resulted in a closer examination of the kind of guidelines managed care programs are using and who is writing these protocols. It is essential that you understand the potential effects of the restrictions that affect the care you may receive and your options for being treated outside the managed care network, as well as other strictures of the utilization management system in your MCO.

You Must Take Charge! Don't Take No for an Answer!

Although it isn't logistically simple, if you're enrolled in a managed care program, you have to take the initiative when organizational restrictions impinge on the quality of your care. This includes taking issue with the utilization managers, who are on the front line and make such decisions as when you may be admitted to the hospital, how long you can stay, and where you can go for what care.

In the managed care system, the decision with regard to how long a patient can remain in the hospital is no longer up to the treating physician. Managed care organizations have developed a variety of practice guidelines that specify the appropriate duration of hospitalization for given diagnoses.

To find out what these guidelines are, check out the National Guideline Clearing House, available through the web at *http://www.guideline.gov.* Currently, more than 300 guidelines have been developed by medical specialty societies, federal agencies, health plans, and hospitals. It is expected that, by the end of 2001, there will be more than 3,500 readily available at this website, which has been funded by the federal government, the American Medical Association, and the American Association of Health Plans.

It is the limitations and restrictions of treatment as established in these guidelines that is the most problematic area for patients who are enrolled in managed care programs. The issue of disallowed care is of major concern. It is clear that this is an area that can lead to litigation when expensive but appropriate interventions are disallowed.

It is the utilization managers, employees of the managed care company, who oversee the implementation of these guidelines. Remember, these utilization managers, or case managers, are not physicians. Sometimes they are nurses who are simply following corporate guidelines, which are based, in large measure, on fiscal considerations. While it is helpful to have some indication of how your own physician feels about any given issue, you must remember that it is now possible for you to be involved in a relationship that has an inherent conflict of interest. Your doctor may not feel free to express an independent opinion. If the response to the question you have raised with the case manager is not satisfactory, you must make clear your dissatisfaction and insist on speaking with one of the company's physicians. Most likely, the first company physician you speak with will adhere to the party line. The next step is to bring your problem to the managed care company's director of medical policy. This individual is commonly the final arbiter within the company in these matters. While it is a cumbersome and hierarchical structure that is inherently difficult to challenge, I want to assure you that there are always exceptions to every rule.

I have lost count of the number of times I had to do battle with managed care organizations over patient care issues that ranged from minute to monumental. The striking thing about each and every one is that, in every instance, the managed care organization caved. I am convinced that my patients, without my aggressive and many times offensive intervention, would not have succeeded had they taken on the system on their own. So it is very important that you have a physician ally when you go into battle with the managed care organization. The most common problems a surgeon encounters in dealing with case managers has to do with hospitalizations. Preoperative stays are often routinely disallowed and the length of postoperative hospital stays are limited. I have also been involved in battles with respect to the need for certain treatments and diagnostic procedures. Certain general principles emerge from these exchanges. Most commonly, I have challenged the utilization manager and fought my way up the chain of command. Recently, I was in a debate with a physician reviewer who was standing firm until I learned that he was a retired psychiatrist. When I challenged his expertise, he was forced to admit that he was relying on the MCO's guideline. It was only after I insisted on speaking with someone I could justifiably consider a peer, a surgeon, that I made any headway and eventually prevailed. In this regard, you should know that in many cases these physician reviewers are the employees of companies contracted by the managed care company to handle medical reviews. In my experience, the fact that approval decisions on treatment is a multilayered corporate process can work to your advantage. But this is only true if your physician is willing to join the battle and insists on dealing with a peer. These battles are all time-consuming, but when faced with my relentless challenge, the authorities have decided that it was the better part of wisdom to allow me to practice medicine without their interference.

While these battles are frequently unpleasant exchanges, in all candor, I always felt that I was dealing with someone whose corporate mandate was no match for a well-informed, motivated physician with a tangible and immediate obligation to a patient.

Like most insurance companies, managed care organizations know that most people are easily intimidated and are not likely to challenge a decision. Because most potential problems do not involve life-or-death issues or dollar amounts that would warrant retaining a lawyer, most patients usually do not question the official interpretation of their contract. If you find any decision unacceptable, the first thing you must do is validate that decision. There is absolutely no reason for you to accept less medical coverage than you paid for or that is provided under your contract.

The next level of dispute, with regard to a difference between what you are being told and what you expect and want, is based on the laws that require every managed care organization to review any medical decision that a patient contends will have an adverse effect on his or her health. If you are not dealing with a medical emergency, some policies have an established grievance review procedure; you should demand a review by the managed care organization's administrative physician. An expedited review can be requested if you or your PCP are dissatisfied with the decision of the managed care company.

Where such a standardized grievance process is not in place, the wisest policy is for you to work your way through the hierarchy within the managed care organization. You must sequentially move up the ladder of responsibility, taking your problem from the case manager to a medical director, then to the senior medical director for policy. At each step along the way you must describe your situation in detail and make it clear that what has been suggested is unacceptable. You should create a paper trail recording the response of each of the employees of the managed care organization with whom you discussed your problem. In addition to bringing your issue to the attention of company officials, you should view this as a fact-finding mission. Commonly, you will find that the organization is willing to revise its decision based on your persistent challenge. If this proves not to be the case, you will have collected the data you need to move the issue to the next level of appeal.

I cringe at the prospect of entering into a substantive contest with a managed care organization. And the problems most commonly involve your choice of a physician, a hospital, or a treatment. While it is true that you are your best advocate, you need allies. First and foremost, your physician must be on your side. If you and your doctor believe that a bone marrow or stem cell transplant with high-dose chemotherapy will give you your best shot at surviving breast cancer or myeloma or non-Hodgkins lymphoma and are willing to take the risks, you, of course, want to go to the facility with the most experience and best results in the treatment. If there is a question about whether your child, who had ten ear infections last winter, should have an operation, you want an otorhinolaryngologist—an ear, nose, and throat specialist—who has had substantial experience operating on children. If you have questions about the best treatment for your prostate cancer and are not sure whether radiation makes more sense for you than surgery, and you want to consult with a radiation oncologist as well as a urologist, and the managed care organization has said no, you must have a doctor on your side who believes you should get what you want. In addition to your physician, you should bring this matter to the attention of your employer and/or the employee benefits program administrator in hopes of getting their support. You can get useful information from the staff in your physician's office—secretaries, aides, nurses—who have had experience dealing with your managed care organization.

If you cannot get your physician to participate in appealing a denial of care, even if it involves an out-of-pocket expense, you should obtain a second opinion consultation in hopes of finding a physician partner who will tackle the managed care bureaucracy.

If all your efforts to negotiate a satisfactory resolution within your managed care organization have been to no avail, you must request the clinical reasons for the denial in writing. You already have a record of the names of the people with whom you have discussed the decision, including their clinical training, background, experience, and official position in the organization. You now have to ask your doctor to provide you with a written explanation of the reasons for recommending the treatment plan. You should also obtain a written report from any physicians you consulted independently.

The managed care organization will have a highly specific document of your case. Your records must match that one in precision and detail. Once this matter is taken outside of the managed care organization, your records are the basis of your appeal. The managed care organization has all the money and lawyers it needs at its disposal. In addition, it has financial incentives to delay even those payments it knows it will have to make in the future. If you do not get satisfaction, and the amount of money in dispute is not too large, you can file a claim in small claims court, where you will not need a lawyer. Once you retain a lawyer to represent you, the company will no longer communicate with you directly.

In this process, you should turn for help to the appropriate information resources and advocacy groups. Such voluntary health agencies as the American Heart Association, Cancer Care, or the American Diabetes Association have established protocols that are the accepted standard of care in many clinical situations. You are entitled to care that meets the standards that have been established by these independent groups with instant prestige as experts. There are many patient advocacy groups that have developed diverse strategies for dealing with individuals involved in disputes with their MCOs. There are many examples, such as breast cancer and AIDS, where the assistance of these advocacy groups has resulted in changes in the decision of a managed care organization with respect to the denial of a treatment. You should write to the state insurance department compliance office detailing the issue concerning the MCO's failure to provide adequate coverage. You should also write similar letters to your elected local, state, and federal political representatives, and copy your MCO. Managed care organizations are famous for changing their position when faced with adverse public or political attention. They are all uniformly unhappy when their actions become the topic of an exposé on evening news programs. No decision that leads to significant embarrassment of the organization will stand. It is an almost automatic response to disown a denial of service when confronted with having to defend a decision that has been publicized and given a real live face.

I don't want to mislead you; if you are forced to go it alone, while I wish you luck, I think your chances of success are slim. With each contact in the managed care organization, you must ask to whom that person reports. Your appeal should then be directed to that person. You must persist and make your way through the hierarchy of the managed care organization after enlisting as many supporters as possible using the information from the independent agencies cited here.

The recent decision of Aetna U.S. Healthcare to create an external review policy for denied coverage decisions is a very encouraging sign. While other managed care companies have external review policies, this is the first case of a national company implementing this practice for all its products and enrollees for all HMO and point-of-service contracts. Under this new program, only after exhausting their internal appeals procedures can a patient or doctor request an external review. The details lead me to believe that it is a very small step, but in the right direction. A cynical view of this move sees it as a means of deferring the imposition of any far-reaching governmental regulations. However, it is encouraging to think that in order to maintain market share in this highly competitive field, Aetna's initiative may result in other managed care companies following suit.

During my short tenure as a part-time senior medical director for policy at Empire Blue Cross/Blue Shield, I was even more distressed by the capricious system for making decisions that was pivotal in the care of a given patient. It was astonishing to me that patients with comparable problems had a given treatment allowed or disallowed not because of the nature of their disease but solely as a result of the judgment of the particular medical director to whom the person was directed. One of the most glaring discrepancies involved the use of such high-tech procedures as bone marrow and stem cell transplants and other treatments that can be claimed to still be under investigation and not of proven merit. This lack of standardization of approved treatment is not uncommon. It is the source of embarrassment for the many managed care organizations who find their lack of uniformity a topic for the nightly local television news, and at the same time provides both physicians and patients with firm grounds when questioning an unacceptable decision. The absence of a standard response is your loophole. Use it.

As I've said, if you question the decision of a case manager, you will normally be shunted to a medical director. You should immediately determine this person's field of expertise and whether he or she has any track record with regard to your problem. If you do not get satisfaction from the medical director, you should ask to speak to the medical director for policy. If this does not result in an acceptable resolution, the next step involves getting opinions through an external review. Most MCOs have outside resources to which they turn when questions are raised in this regard. These are the extramural reviewers they use as authorities in such instances. You are entitled to know the basis and the source for any decision with regard to these issues.

It is the customary lack of their uniform application of policy, as delineated in their practice guidelines, that allows patients to win their battles. It is striking just how often a persistent patient ultimately gets permission to obtain care from a nonparticipating physician or at a noncooperating institution. Time and again, I have been impressed with the fact that it is indeed the squeaky wheel that is allowed to have a stem cell transplant or breast reconstruction after initially being told that these treatments were not covered.

In order for you to be able to pursue your best interests, I must emphasize once again that it is vital for you to maintain a complete and detailed written record of everyone you talk to with regard to your coverage and payment for your care. Take notes for every phone conversation and date them; after these conversations send confirming letters to the managed care company and to your physician. Keep copies of everything you write and a meticulous record of every contact.

How to Lodge a Complaint

- Discuss any potential problem with your PCP and have a full discussion concerning the options and the recommendations.
- If you have any doubts about your options, ask for a written report from your doctor and obtain a second opinion.
- If there are differences between the two physicians, discuss them with your PCP or specialist.
- When these issues are resolved, if a question arises with the managed care organization with regard to coverage, discuss these with a case manager.

- Ask for and obtain a written report from the case manager.
- With the cooperation of your PCP or specialist, move your unresolved issues up the chain of command in the managed care organization.
- Keep meticulous written records every step of the way.
- Request an external review.
- Understand that every final decision is based on a negotiated settlement that can take time and involve substantial effort on your part to get the care you want and need.

Liability

One of the most troublesome issues with regard to managed care involves the question of liability for malpractice over decisions to deny and decisions to delay treatment, or to direct medical management through the use of guidelines prepared by the managed care company and issued to its participating physicians. This highly charged issue has been joined by patients and organized medicine and is the pivotal argument in the debate about how far government should go in regulating managed care. It has become the subject of an intensive lobbying effort.

The arguments that have been raised by the managed care companies against holding them legally accountable are based on the claim that this will increase the cost of litigation and, in turn, the cost of their liability insurance. They also suggest that consumers will solve quality issues by "voting with their feet." In addition, they are quick to point out that the courts are currently allowing some malpractice suits.

Most consumers are severely limited in suing their health plans over coverage decisions. This is a result of a 1974 federal law known as the Employee Retirement Income Security Act (ERISA), which regulates employer-sponsored health plans. This law, as most commonly interpreted, prohibits patients who have been injured as a result of coverage denials from suing employer-sponsored plans in state court for lost wages, pain and suffering, or punitive damages. They can only sue in federal court for the cost of the benefit that was not approved.

Health care plans are vigorously defending their position, which allows them to regulate utilization while at the same time denying responsibility if something goes wrong. They have received some support from employers who are concerned that they may end up being held liable for decisions made by their health plans. With claims that lawyers rather than patients will benefit from any changes in the existing limitations for litigation, since it is employers and insurers who will be viewed as having far deeper pockets than physicians, they have become natural allies in the upcoming battle over responsibility.

On the other side of the argument are consumer groups and physicians, who have had their autonomy over clinical decisions eroded by the managed care plans. They argue that making it easier to sue health plans for coverage will make the health plans accountable for bad decisions, since the threat alone of litigation may result in improvement in the quality of care. This is a contest that has just begun and will be fought state by state. While it remains to be seen if the current legal restrictions will be overridden or revised, eventually this issue may well be brought to the Supreme Court. It is important that you know your rights and options as of now.

In Massachusetts recently, a woman with breast cancer challenged the decision of her HMO to deny her a bone marrow transplant; they instead prescribed a less expensive course of chemotherapy. The patient claimed that denying the transplant was an economic decision. The court determined that the woman's charges constituted a malpractice claim that was not superceded by the federal ERISA laws. In this case, the physicians were employed directly by the HMO and the court concluded that therefore the HMO had committed malpractice. Since the plan covered all "medically necessary treatments," the court ruled that there was no difference between a physician's responsibility to render treatment consistent with "standard of care" rules and the provision of "medically necessary" treatments. The woman had her bone marrow transplant.

Cracks are forming in the walls of the ERISA fortress that may well result in health care plans being held liable for the decisions they make. In 1997, Texas passed the first law giving patients the right to sue HMOs for medical malpractice. The appeal of this decision by Aetna U.S. Healthcare was rejected in the federal courts. In Pennsylvania, the state supreme court ruled that an HMO cannot claim an exemption based on the ERISA statutes. Two states, Texas and Massachusetts, have passed legislative initiatives that permit their citizens to challenge a managed care company in court on the basis of alleged medical malpractice. Several state courts have held that where managed care plans inject themselves into the clinical decisions that affect the quality of care, there must be the potential for legal remedy. In California, Aetna U.S. Healthcare was held liable in a benefits denial case and $116 million in punitive damages was awarded to the plaintiff. Judgments with large awards will have a profound effect in the very near future of making the ERISA-covered plans more accountable.

Hold On to Your Medical Record: You Paid for It and It Protects You

You own your medical records, including all X-rays and laboratory results and reports. In order to maintain the integrity and accessibility of these records, you need to hold on to them.

David Solomon is an executive with severe leg pain whose slipped disk had been missed in the initial CAT scan (the full story is discussed later). The second scan uncovered the problem and he underwent spinal surgery. The second scan, in addition to his slipped disk, also revealed an abnormality in his left hip. The radiologist was concerned. Privately, he told me that he thought it might represent a cancer in the bone. After a brief discussion, David agreed to have a biopsy done, which indicated a benign bone cyst.

Ten years later, David Solomon, now sixty-five years old, was having his annual executive physical examination. He had an abnormal blood test that was interpreted to be consistent with prostate cancer. An appropriate workup was done. The defect in his left hip showed up on the new CAT scan and on the bone scan. Now, since Solomon didn't have the films of the scan that had been done ten years earlier, the bone scan was interpreted as being consistent with a metastasis from his prostate cancer, which would mean that he was not a candidate for prostate surgery. If he had the old X-rays and/or the slides of the biopsy done ten years earlier, his current physicians could have ignored this abnormal finding. And so, once again, Solomon had to go through the discomfort and accept the inherent risks of a bone biopsy.

The lesson here is simple: Your medical record is extremely valuable. You cannot count on any institution to maintain your records as carefully and as faithfully as you can yourself. Any part of that record may become important at some future date. Be sure when you have X-rays taken that you secure a copy for your own files. There is usually a modest charge for duplicating your records, and it will not be covered by insurance. Pay it anyway! If at any time you are found to have a mass noted on a mammogram or an unusual shadow on a chest X-ray or a lesion on a CAT scan, these previous films will play a significant role in determining what will be done in the face of a new finding.

Keep an orderly medical record that includes the results of all laboratory tests and copies of any and all operative reports and hospital discharge summaries. There is no way of predicting when these files will be important or even vital to future decisions concerning your medical care. Having them close at hand will help you wage any battles with your MCO over treatments and liability.

CHAPTER 2

Getting the Right Doctor

R egardless of how you look at medical care, the doctor is the unquestioned dominant force. He or she dwarfs every other element in the process. You may have an idealized notion of the doctor you want; a skilled, sensitive, selfless, dedicated physician who will care for you and about you. While this description was on target for many generations, that kind of doctor is a vanishing breed, placed on the list of endangered species as a result of the hostile environment of managed care, where the very traits you so value prohibit a doctor's chance to thrive and are, in many ways, actively discouraged.

If you are one of the millions of Americans now enrolled in a managed care program, you were probably handed a provider directory, one of the hefty insignia of "new era" medicine. This is the managed care enrollee's bible, the listing of the physicians and nonphysician providers who have agreed and are under contract to participate in your plan. When you screwed up your courage and first opened this telephone-directory-size, bare-bones list of names, addresses, and telephone numbers, you probably looked first to see if the names of your physician or gynecologist and your child's pediatrician were listed. If you didn't see them, with a sigh of resignation and a shrug of bewilderment, you probably searched for the name of physicians from your hometown or immediate neighborhood. In other words, you decided convenience was the most important qualification for your doctor. Unfortunately, a physician's office location is a very poor predictor of professional adequacy, let alone excellence. What should you be looking for?

All Doctors Are Not Created Equal

The public has bought the myth, promoted by the medical profession, that the medical mistakes they hear about in the media are the result of bad doctors. There are, without a doubt, incompetent and unethical physicians who are sued and/or lose their license to practice medicine. However, all doctors make mistakes. Every surgeon, even the best of them, makes one, two, three, or more mistakes, some very serious, every year. They just don't tell you or me about them. I know; I was one of them. Every year, 120,000 or so people die as a result of the care they have received. So, bad things can happen to patients with the best doctors. There is, however, no question that bad things happen much more frequently to patients who have bad doctors. You have to recognize that there is a difference.

Before the end of most consultations, my patients often tell me, "I came to you, Dr. Barron, because I know you are the best." Early in my career I accepted these comments uncritically. They were, after all, enormously ego-satisfying. It took a while before I recognized this compliment as nothing more than the expression of a deeply felt wish on the part of patients that they had put themselves in the hands of a competent physician.

The truth is doctors know that, in almost all fields of medicine, with very, very, very few exceptions, this is a myth; there is no "best." Much more frightening is the widespread silent acceptance by physicians that the variation in the quality of care delivered by their colleagues is enormous, and that the level of care provided to the average person can be very far below standard.

A recent study carried out in Louisiana demonstrated that more than 40 percent of patients died as a result of advanced cancer that had remained undetected and therefore untreated prior to their deaths. This is stark evidence that even though we live in the era of CAT scans and other high-technology medicine, significant medical problems go unrecognized. This study provides a graphic demonstration of the astonishing variability in the competence of practicing physicians.

So, putting first things first, it is vital that you recognize that the real differences among physicians are enormous. This is true even among those with apparently identical credentials.

> The first article of the Declaration of the Informed Medical Consumer is: "All doctors are not created equal."

What Does My Doctor Know and How, Where, and When Did He or She Learn It?

Medical School

The vast majority of physicians in the United States are graduates of American and Canadian medical schools or schools of osteopathic medicine. They have had a striking uniformity in their training that typically involves four years of medical school. A lockstep program of courses in the basic medical sciences is followed by two years of clinical clerkships in medicine, surgery, pediatrics, obstetrics and gynecology, and the other fields of medicine where student doctors get their initial exposure to the care of patients. For all intents and purposes, there are essentially no significant differences in the training provided to the students of these institutions.

This is not true of American graduates of foreign medical schools and non-Americans who attend medical schools outside of North America or Western Europe. As a rule, their training usually deviates markedly from the quality that has been established by medical school accrediting bodies in both the United States and Canada.

I have been impressed by the fact that, regardless of the school they attended, there is an astonishingly small difference among the best medical students at North American schools. This, however, is not true for those not at or close to the top of their class. And in the lower regions of class ranks, the differences can be scary. However, regardless of what medical school a student has attended, there is almost uniform agreement among knowledgeable physicians that it is entirely possible for a mediocre medical student who graduates from a North American medical school to become an outstanding practicing physician.

I have an example from my own experience that highlights the defect in predicting just who will become a good physician. In the late 1960s, the competition for admission to every medical school in the United States was very keen. At the time, there were six medical schools in New York City. A young man who had been rejected from every one of the twelve schools to which he had applied came to New York

City on the first of September and called the admissions office at each medical school. His message was "I'm here. If someone you have accepted doesn't turn up or has changed his or her mind about going to medical school, I'm ready to take that person's place." As it turned out, one school had such an unanticipated vacancy. Although the dean of admissions knew the school could fill the empty slot by going to their waiting list, that would be logistically difficult and time-consuming. For administrative reasons alone, this student, who had been rejected by the medical school in question, found that his initiative landed him in the freshman class. He graduated in the middle of the class and is today, from all reports, a respected physician in his community.

Each year approximately 16,000 students begin and an almost equal number are graduated from the 122 medical schools in the United States. It is, in fact, almost impossible to flunk out of medical school today. This is true whether you are a student at Harvard, one of the oldest and most prestigious medical schools in the country, or at the East Tennessee State University James H. Quillen School of Medicine, one of the newest.

There is a standing joke among medical students that goes: Question: What do you call the person who's at the bottom of the class on graduation day? Answer: "Doctor!" Since medical training is a cumulative process, it is possible, though unlikely, that someone at the bottom of a class will be able to move into the top ranks in his or her chosen field. Should you ask a prospective doctor what his or her class rank was? I'd skip it. It is, however, worth finding out where he or she went to medical school, since everything else being equal, you will most probably be better served by a physician trained in North America. You have heard the names of the great universities—Harvard, Yale, Columbia,

Stanford, Duke, Vanderbilt, Michigan, McGill. They all have first-class medical schools. I wouldn't choose a doctor solely because he or she had attended a top-rated medical school, but I would give him or her the edge. There are some lesser medical schools in North America, but their product is still uniformly better than the doctors trained in Eastern Europe or the Indian subcontinent. This is not xenophobia. It is recognition of the real differences that exist among the training programs for physicians in different parts of the world.

Residency Training, Teaching Hospitals, Academic Medical Centers

Medical school is most commonly followed by what is referred to as residency. Most residencies begin on July 1 each year, and the current designations for residents are PGY1, PGY2, and so on, which refers to the postgraduate year of training. Doctors in the first postgraduate year, PGY1, are sometimes called interns. Residency programs are organized by and take place in what are known as "teaching hospitals."

The most prestigious residency programs, which attract the best medical school graduates, are closely associated with medical schools in what are known as university or university-affiliated hospitals. The combination of a medical school and its affiliated hospital is known as an academic medical center.

Which is the best medical school? Where is the best residency? There's no simple answer to these questions. The medical school of any major university is most commonly a first-class institution. Harvard, Yale, Duke, Columbia, Johns Hopkins, Stanford, University of Chicago, Georgetown, Pennsylvania, and Texas are universities with excellent medical

schools and there are another ten or so of essentially equivalent eminence, including Virginia, Cornell, Northwestern,
Michigan, North Carolina, Washington University in St.
Louis, Vanderbilt, McGill in Canada, Emory, and the University of California at San Francisco.

With regard to residency training, it is inappropriate to
attempt to rank institutions, since the appropriate focus
needs to be much sharper and better-defined, on a specific
clinical specialty. If you need a cardiac surgeon, it is of little import that the institution can boast three world-class
neurologists. The excellence of a department is basically
a function of the chairman or clinical director, the senior
clinicians that staff the department, and the patients who
are attracted by the competence and achievements of the
physicians. Superstar physicians are very much like superstar athletes; they often move from place to place with dizzying speed. Hospitals will pay the equivalent of a large signing
bonus to a world-class expert in reproductive endocrinology
who will attract infertile patients whose treatment will generate millions of dollars of revenue for the institution. A
prestigious pediatric cardiac surgeon can bring in a sufficient amount of money to support the research efforts of an
entire department of pediatrics. So asking for the "best" department of surgery or pediatrics is taking aim at a moving
target.

Residency Training Positions—A Buyer's Market

There are more than 7,500 residency programs in the
United States with more than 34,000 PGY1 positions that are
approved and continually evaluated by one of the twenty-
four different American Boards of Medical Specialties (ABMS).
So there are more than two PGY1 residency positions for
every one of the 16,000 graduates of American medical

schools. The graduates of foreign medical schools are placed in the vast majority of the residency positions not filled by graduates of American medical schools.

Physician Training—
A Function of Good Teachers and Good Patients

As with all apprenticeships, students in the third and fourth year of medical school, known as clinical clerks, and residents are dependent upon their *teachers* and what they can learn from the illnesses of the *patients* they encounter during their training. Consideration of these two pivotal variables reveals why physicians can complete their medical education and harbor massive gaps in their medical knowledge and technical abilities. Not every hospital or medical school can boast a teaching faculty of the caliber of such prestigious institutions as Stanford or Johns Hopkins. Nor is it as likely that a patient with a rare disease such as a pro-lactin-secreting tumor of the pituitary gland will be found in Peoria, Illinois, as at the Columbia-Presbyterian Medical Center in New York City.

While it is difficult to accept and runs counter to the wishes and assumptions of patients, the quality of medical education is not dependent on a rigorous system of passing the art and science of medicine from one generation to another. Few hospitals, even university-affiliated ones, offer formal structured training for the resident staff. In large measure, the hospital ward is the focal center of medical training with the youngest member of the medical team instructed by the one who has just finished his or her own first year of residency. This method of training physicians materially affects the quality of patient care. There is a saying often repeated by doctors in training, "See one, do one, teach one." In many cases, this is not much of an exaggeration. You should remember and recall this regrettably all-too-true aphorism when you are hospitalized and find that your care is delegated to a doctor-in-training.

Another significant issue in the training of physicians, medical students, and residents alike is the rapidly changing management of a significant spectrum of diseases. Many acute diseases of the past such as diphtheria and tetanus are now preventable and rarely seen. Doctors-in-training will more likely have to treat emergent conditions, such as heart attacks and stroke, for which effective interventions have recently been developed. While there is general agreement in the profession that up-to-the-minute training can make a big difference in a patient's welfare, it's not clear that there has been an appropriate response and modification of the training of physicians. (In the chapters on hospitals and procedures, there is a detailed discussion of the effects of this system on patients and how to defend yourself when you are in need of such care and in the hands of an amateur in a teaching hospital.)

As in medical school, the progressive promotion of residents, even the less competent and incompetent, is standard practice. In our current litigious environment, in many instances, the system, when faced with weak residents, many of whom may have been undeservedly graduated from medical school, is dissuaded from action as a result of the threat of possible legal action by the trainee whom they could rightfully dismiss. This allows the resident to transfer to a different program without adverse information concerning his or her faults being transmitted to the training program into which he or she is being accepted. These marginal doctors eventually enter unsupervised private practice where there is little effective control to protect their patients.

Perhaps the most dramatic evidence of the lack of

equality in residency training programs has been the recent acknowledgment by the Accreditation Council for Graduate Medical Education (ACGME) of the need to include educational outcomes assessment in the residency review process. This represents the candid acceptance of the need not only to know whether a training program provides residents with adequate opportunities to learn but also to ascertain whether a program's residents actually develop into competent physicians.

It is the ACGME organization that is responsible for evaluating the quality of residency programs. Traditionally, accreditation reviews have not tackled the more difficult task of evaluating outcomes. It has been widely recognized by the medical accrediting bodies that knowledge, skills, attitudes, and professionalism are very difficult to measure. I know it will be a shock to you but there is currently no existing rigorous attempt to evaluate these fundamental characteristics of newly trained physicians except through tests designed to demonstrate clinical knowledge and cognitive skills but not clinical performance. The ACGME is now initiating research programs in order to determine how this can best be accomplished.

The Color-Blind Surgeon with a Tremor

At one point in my career, a resident was admitted to the program who, although he was intellectually up to the task, had an unfortunate tremor. This would have been of no consequence had he chosen a medical specialty that did not require manual dexterity, hand-eye coordination, and depth perception. Although it is difficult to believe, there is to my knowledge no surgical residency program that tests applicants for these critical traits, which, I am convinced, if not inborn are almost impossible to teach.

I had not had any contact with this particular resident until the middle of his second year of training. We were working in the operating room together for the first time when I noticed this singular disability for a surgeon. His hand shook. Knowing my reputation among the residents as being somewhat of a tyrant, I at first thought he was nervous simply because he was working with me. I tried to put him at ease. Although I complimented him on his performance, things didn't improve, and since we had a long and difficult case ahead of us, I decided to confront the issue and asked, "Am I making you nervous?"

"Oh no, Dr. Barron. Not at all. That's not it. I have a tremor," he admitted.

I was aghast. There was no alternative other than to continue. I took complete charge and let him do nothing of consequence. I didn't even trust him to tie sutures properly. We finished the operation. For the benefit of all my patients, I want to assure you the patient did well.

At the end of the day I went to the chairman's office to register my opinion that this young man should be encouraged to find some other line of work. Just as I began my argument, the chairman held up his hand and said, "I know exactly what you are going to say. I know he is color-blind, but there are many good surgeons who have that problem."

This is not a joke. Today, out there in America, is a color-blind surgeon with a tremor who completed a residency in a surgical subspecialty at a top-notch institution.

The number of mediocre and outright incompetent residents is not small. While the best graduates of the best medical schools are admitted to the best residency programs, those of lesser skill and demonstrated ability who are desperately in need of the best training are relegated to lesser hospitals, where their own inadequacies are most often further amplified by inadequate supervision and training. This chain reaction is what makes and perpetuates the great medical institutions of our country, but it is, ultimately, a disservice to the community, since at the same time it results in the continued output of physicians who by virtue of their limited training and experience provide medical care of lesser quality.

Fortunately, most physicians are rarely required to provide care to the seriously ill. The vast majority of medical care is provided by practicing physicians who see three different groups of patients: ambulatory patients with self-limiting illnesses that in the essentially healthy person will resolve with or without medical intervention; patients with chronic diseases who are in stable condition without acute problems; and what we call "the worried well." While these patients require advice and counsel, patience and reassurance, the resolution or progress of their medical problems is usually not materially affected by the quality of the medical care they receive.

It is the medical student, resident, and hospital-based physician who most frequently care for the really sick patients, those with acute emergent conditions including heart attacks and stroke, asthmatics in respiratory distress, accident victims and those who are hemorrhaging; patients in diabetic coma or with such complications of that disease as blindness, kidney failure, and gangrene of a foot; the patient with gallstones awaiting surgery; the patient with end-stage ovarian cancer. These are the physicians on the front line in the care of patients with significant illness or in medical crises.

Board Certification—
Credentialing Following Residency

Although doctors with a medical license issued by a state government can establish themselves in practice in any specialty, board certification by one of the American Board of Medical Specialties (ABMS) is the basic credential of physician competence in a medical specialty. The provider directory of many managed care organizations includes the designation "board-certified" for those participating physicians who have this credential.

After completing a formal, structured residency program that ranges from three to seven years in length, most certifying specialty boards require an additional period of independent patient-care experience before permitting physicians to take the required examinations that will result in their being "board-certified."

Until comparatively recently, taking the examinations for board certification was a once-in-a-lifetime exercise for a physician. Now, most specialty boards certify a physician for a fixed period of time and require periodic reexamination and reevaluation for recertification for an additional term. There have been substantial debates within the profession that these exams are not designed to demonstrate competence as a practicing physician. Claims have been made that recertification exams are, as currently structured, not adequate for weeding out incompetents. People have come to equate, for lack of any other measure, board certification with competence since it is one of the few accessible indicators that they have. Since initial certification is attained close to the end of the applicant's formal training, which is presumably up-to-the-minute, it is by its very nature a better index of a doctor's competency than any subsequent recertification exam that may be required by the specialty board.

However, there is no doubt that as physicians become more and more remote from their formal training, this credential is of decreasing value.

Beyond residency training, there are additional formal structured programs in many specialties, known as fellowships, that can lead to an additional qualification in a subspecialty. For example, a doctor who has completed a residency in internal medicine may choose to take additional training in cardiology, gastroenterology, endocrinology, or pulmonary medicine. One who has completed a surgical residency may go on to a fellowship in cardiothoracic surgery. There are literally dozens of such subspecialty programs. Almost all boards that approve residency programs and govern standards in each specialty have one or more subspecialties in which a physician may be credentialed.

The complexity of the structure of specialty and subspecialty credentialing is demonstrated in the following table.

MEDICAL SPECIALTIES AND SUBSPECIALTIES

AMERICAN BOARDS	SUBSPECIALTIES
Allergy and Immunology	Diagnostic Laboratory Immunology
Anesthesiology	Critical Care Medicine Pain Management
Colon and Rectal Surgery	
Dermatology	Dermatopathology Cutaneous Micrographic Surgery Dermatologic Immunology
Emergency Medicine	Sports Medicine Pediatric Emergency Medicine
Family Practice	Geriatric Medicine Sports Medicine
Internal Medicine	Adolescent Medicine Cardiac Electrophysiology Cardiovascular Disease Critical Care Medicine Diagnostic Laboratory Immunology Endocrinology and Metabolism Gastroenterology Geriatric Medicine Hematology Infectious Disease Oncology Nephrology Pulmonary Disease Rheumatology Sports Medicine
Medical Genetics	
Neurological Surgery	Critical Care Medicine
Nuclear Medicine	Nuclear Radiology Radioisotopic Pathology
Obstetrics and Gynecology	Gynecologic Oncology Maternal and Fetal Medicine Reproductive Endocrinology Critical Care Medicine
Ophthalmology	
Orthopedic Surgery	Hand Surgery
Otolaryngology	Pediatric Otolaryngology

AMERICAN BOARDS	SUBSPECIALTIES
Pathology	Blood Banking
	Chemical Pathology
	Cytopathology
	Dermatopathology
	Forensic Pathology
	Hematology
	Immunopathology
	Medical Microbiology
	Neuropathology
	Pediatric Pathology
	Radioisotopic Pathology
Pediatrics	Adolescent Medicine
	Pediatric Cardiology
	Pediatric Critical Care Medicine
	Pediatric Endocrinology
	Pediatric Emergency Medicine
	Pediatric Gastroenterology
	Pediatric Hematology-Oncology
	Pediatric Infectious Disease
	Pediatric Immunology
	Pediatric Nephrology
	Pediatric Pulmonology
	Pediatric Rheumatology
	Pediatric Sports Medicine
	Neo-natal Perinatal Medicine
Physical Medicine and Rehabilitation	
Plastic Surgery	
Preventive Medicine	Undersea Medicine
	Medical Toxicology
Psychiatry and Neurology	Addition Psychiatry
	Child and Adolescent Psychiatry
	Geriatric Psychiatry
	Clinical Neurophysiology
Radiology	Nuclear Radiology
	Radiation Oncology
	Neuroradiology
	Pediatric Radiology
	Interventional Radiology
Surgery	Vascular Surgery
	Hand Surgery
	Surgical Critical Care
	Pediatric Surgery
Thoracic Surgery	
Urology	

Everything else being equal, you want a doctor who

- graduated from a medical school in North America. The more well known the school with a reputation for excellence the better.
- completed an accredited residency program at a highly regarded academic medical center.
- is certified by the appropriate specialty board.
- has been in practice for three or more years.
- has admitting privileges at an excellent hospital where you would choose to be treated.

You should obtain all these data prior to your visit to a doctor's office. Ask the physician's staff when making the first appointment. While much of the important information about the physicians who participate in a managed care program is not included in your provider directory, some of it is readily available in the *Directory of Medical Specialists*. This is a listing of all currently active board-certified physicians; it includes the details of a doctor's training, professional experience, specialty credentials, and hospital affiliations. A current edition of this book is available in most public libraries and this data is available on the internet at *www.certifieddoctor.org*. The American Medical Association database, *www.ama-assn.org*, has much of the same information about its members.

The second article of the Declaration of the Informed Medical Consumer is: "I must know what my doctor knows and how, where, and when he or she learned it."

Specialty Societies, Medical Clubs, Wanna-be Specialties

In addition to the constituent boards of the American Boards of Medical Specialties that credential specialists and subspecialists, there are more than eighty American Medical Association specialty societies that physicians can join that reflect their more focused special medical interests, and almost five hundred different training programs creating even more subdivisions of existing specialties and subspecialties. For example, an orthopedic surgeon may choose to take special training in shoulder surgery, knee surgery, hip replacement, or endoscopic joint surgery.

Many of these subspecialists are not formally approved, have no specific credential by the specialty board, or are newly developed programs that have been established in the hope of one day receiving formal accreditation from the relevant specialty board. This multitiered training and certification process contributes to the complexity of evaluating any doctor's training.

You should be alert to the fact that many of the certificates that line the walls of your doctor's office may attest simply to participation in a continuing medical education course. Continuing medical education is a very, very big lucrative business that provides the doctor with the opportunity, for example, to take a tax-deductible cruise to some exotic spot while attending two two-hour lecture sessions aboard ship every day or to enjoy a week of skiing at Aspen or Sun Valley with lectures given before and at the end of each day on the slopes, also with the lion's share of the cost of this working vacation being tax-deductible.

The often impressive-looking certificates of attendance distributed at the conclusion of one of these jaunts may reflect very little substance with respect to a physician's abilities. If they are on display on the wall, it is a good idea to ask the doctor about them. The answers will give you some insight into this particular form of self-promotion and inject some truth into this kind of advertising.

Admitting Privileges

Admitting privileges to a hospital are a certification that the hospital has determined the physician qualified to practice in that institution. A physician who has admitting privileges is an "attending physician" on the hospital staff. Some physicians will never need to hospitalize patients, but the vast majority do. Without admitting privileges at a specific hospital, your physician can take no active role in your care if and when you are hospitalized.

Most hospitals award admitting privileges very carefully. The most prestigious institutions are the most restrictive and rigorous in their policies. For specialists who do procedures, an application for privileges requires a detailed listing of those procedures they intend to perform and for which they are requesting approval. The responsibility for approving these applications rests with the director of the service and usually requires the agreement of the hospital's chief medical officer. This process is in place because hospitals want the reputation of having only the most highly qualified physicians as members of their staff and at the same time minimize their risk of exposure to medical malpractice suits.

While there is tremendous variability in the requirements that different hospitals have for those applying for privileges, it is important to recognize that all hospitals are now under enormous financial pressure to keep their beds full, and economic forces are playing an increasing role in this decision-making process. In many regions of the country, legislative initiatives now require hospitals to award privileges to almost any willing and able provider. This means that any appropriately licensed physician can apply for privileges.

There are in many institutions prefix modifiers to the title of "attending physician" that include assistant, associate, senior, and consulting. These reflect an ascending hierarchy in the relative seniority of a doctor. This may or may not correlate with the physician's clinical expertise in the management of your particular problem. I have known many instances where a very accomplished surgeon for a specific problem has had a junior title that did not reflect his or her skills and accomplishments.

Medical School Faculty Appointments

The stratification of medical school faculty titles is even more byzantine. In ascending order of rank are instructors, assistant professors, associate professors, and finally professors. Each of these titles can be further modified with prefixes or suffixes that again denote a ranking. The suffix title, for example, professor of clinical medicine—or surgery or obstetrics and gynecology—is usually more prestigious than the prefixed title clinical professor. The unmodified titles, no prefix or suffix, in many medical schools are usually limited to those physicians who dedicate a substantial portion of their time to research.

In any event, there is enormous variability with regard to the meaning of all these insignia of rank from institution to institution. However, a medical school faculty appointment regardless of rank does indicate that a physician is subjected to some additional oversight and professional review.

Honorary Society Memberships

Membership and fellowship in honorary societies are another indication of the status of a physician as measured by his or her peers. There are many medical organizations that a physician may join simply by paying the required dues. And there are others where honorary membership reflects the judgment of those in the field and indicates an individual has made a significant contribution that justifies the special recognition.

A Doctor's Vital Signs—Training and Learning by Experience

There are doctors who have had excellent training but limited clinical experience. This may be due to their junior status or to other aspects of their medical practice. On the other hand, while an older physician may have more experience in treating a given illness, the younger physician may have had more formal training and experience in the use of newer approaches, methods, and technologies.

There is a vast body of literature showing that physicians with substantial experience have a lower complication rate than those with less experience. This is especially important when one is considering undergoing a procedure that is relatively new or involves a recently introduced technology.

Recently, John Cardinal O'Connor of the New York Archdiocese of the Catholic Church was asked to bless a new instrument that had been purchased by the New York University Medical Center for use in the treatment of brain tumors. Although the instrument was anointed by his eminence, and while his blessing is no doubt of substantial value, the natural and critical questions that arise in such a situation are: Who trained the doctor who is going to do the procedure and use this new instrument for the first time at the hospital? How many cases has he or she done and under whose supervision? What does the rest of the staff in this hospital know about the use of the instrument? How have they been trained in its use and in the management of complications that could occur in a patient after it is used?

Primary Care Physicians—The Gatekeepers

Primary care has been officially defined by the Institute of Medicine, an arm of the National Academy of Science in Washington, D.C., as "the provision of integrated accessible health care services by clinicians who are accountable for addressing a large majority of personal health needs, developing a sustained partnership with patients, and practicing in the context of family and community." This has become a core element of the recent redefinition of the field of medicine and the development of what is known as managed care.

The ambitious definition of the responsibilities of the primary care physician highlights its flaws. The PCP is assigned the responsibility of promoting good health, preventing disease and disability, detecting and treating common health problems, educating and counseling patients, and referring patients to other resources when indicated. This involves an exhausting list of tasks; physical examinations; assessment and evaluation of minor acute illness such as colds, infections, and minor traumatic injuries; advice on managing such common conditions as flu, ear infections, and the like; providing prescriptions for medication as well as care instructions, family planning, maternity care for women having normal pregnancies and uncomplicated vaginal deliveries; counseling on health-related behavior;

and perhaps most significantly, the identification of conditions that require referral to more specialized professionals
together with referral to those physicians.

Operationally, primary care means medical practice in
the context of everyday life, distinct and apart from hospital-
based care. The primary care physician is the doctor to
whom patients should turn for care of simple, uncomplicated illness. It is the PCP who by virtue of training, experience, and interest can handle close to 90 percent of the
problems that inspire you to call the doctor.

There are, however, limits to the generalists' capabilities. For example, their training and experience limits their
ability to identify significant medical problems as rapidly as
a specialist. And as a result of their training, they are less
qualified to treat these problems. This is not a trivial difference, and it means that you have to take an active role when
dealing with your PCP in order to minimize the likelihood
that a significant problem is overlooked. One third of PCPs
report that the scope of care they are asked to provide has
increased during the past two years. Twenty-four percent say
they are currently expected to provide a scope of care they
feel is beyond the limits of their competence.

It should be recognized that fiscal concerns led to the
establishment of the primary care model as the mechanism
for containing the costs of medical care, which were being driven, in large measure, by subspecialization and increasing medical technology. These economic forces have
resulted in the primary care provider having a very comprehensive mandate and great responsibility and authority in
the medical care system. The PCP model is also presumed to
be a more patient-friendly approach in the delivery of care.
While it is no doubt less expensive, no one has proven that
cheaper medical care is better care. It has yet to be shown

that this results in any improvement in measurable outcomes while simultaneously decreasing the cost of care.

Who's Who of PCPs

By convention, primary care physicians are trained in
one of the four specialties: family practice, general internal
medicine, pediatrics, or obstetrics and gynecology. Given
the responsibilities and mandate the patient assigns to the
primary care physician, it is essential to recognize the profound differences in training and experience among them.

The general internist and the pediatrician, although
specialists by training, have become generalists caring for
essentially healthy adults and children, respectively, as well
as those with simple illnesses. In the process, they have become competitors of the family practitioner. The American College of Physicians, with support from the American
Board of Internal Medicine, has been spending substantial
amounts of money on advertising in order to maintain the
internists' market share: "So when it's time to choose a
doctor, consider choosing a Doctor of Internal Medicine.
They're the doctors for adults. And whatever else you are,
you're not a kid anymore. For more information, contact a
Doctor of Internal Medicine in your community, or visit our
web site at www.acponline.org." Notwithstanding their advertising, general internal medicine has become a ghetto for
patients who do not fit into one of that specialty's sixteen
"elite" subspecialties. Usually, it is only when a problem in
their narrow field is diagnosed that the super-specialists
in internal medicine have any real interest. For example, a
gastroenterologist will be happy to see a patient with ulcer-
ative colitis or Crohn's disease but is relatively disinterested
in the patient with an upset stomach.

Pediatric office practice primarily involves routine examinations of well babies and children. Again, driven in no small part by economic motives, pediatricians have defined good care as monthly visits during the first year of life, four visits during the child's second year of life, checkups every six months until age six, and yearly visits from then on.

The debate over the requisite skills necessary for providing this care has now been joined by pediatric nurse practitioners. This group of nonphysician health care providers feel that, by virtue of their advanced specialized nursing training, they are appropriately trained to care for well infants and children. It is important to recognize that there is an emphasis on the word *well* here. The argument can be made that so long as there is no evidence of any problem, the nurse practitioner is an appropriate provider of screening health care. I would be very wary of extending this support for the care of any sick child, or one who appears to be deviating in any way from normal in growth, development, or behavior; nurses do not have the extensive medical training of physicians. The professional organizations of pediatricians are now engaged in vociferously defending their own financial self-interest against the claims of their nonphysician nurse colleagues.

Until recently, the family practitioner was at the bottom of the status ladder in the academic medical center. In fact, many academic medical centers have not as yet even established departments of family practice. The differences between the training of a family practitioner and a generalist in internal medicine, both of whom qualify as primary care physicians, are easily identified. The board-certified family practitioner will have spent some time rotating through all the general clinical services, including pediatrics and obstetrics, while internists as a rule usually have had none of these exposures during their residency training. In contrast, there is a very circumscribed focus with regard to the spectrum of disease in the residency training of an obstetrician-gynecologist. Yet physicians in all three of these areas can play the role of primary care provider. In order to preserve their income, some family practitioners have branched out and are now practicing obstetrics and doing minor surgery. All these factors have led to turf wars among members of these different disciplines. Patients must be cautious or they run a risk of getting caught in the cross fire and receiving substandard medical care.

The decision to designate obstetrics and gynecology as a primary care specialty was driven primarily by the fact that the majority of women between the ages of twenty and fifty in urban America identify an obstetrician-gynecologist as their only doctor. The American College of Obstetrics and Gynecology recognized that the burgeoning managed care programs would save money through the primary care gate-keeper system and the imposition of financial disincentives on the primary care physician for referring patients to specialists. Yet this would restrict a patient's access to specialist care and to the technological services that a specialist might recommend. An additional significant motivating force behind the drive to be designated as a primary care specialty was the recognition that the falling birth rate and longer life expectancy are demographic changes that will have a significant effect on the practice of obstetrics and gynecology. In fact, there are very few conditions, diagnoses, or procedures for which obstetrician-gynecologists are the unique provider. In view of the implications of a primary care delivery system model on their practices and income, the professional organizations of obstetricians and gynecologists recognized the imperative to be included among those judged rightful claimants for the role of PCP. They mobilized a very effective and eventually successful political lobbying effort.

The choice of an ob-gyn as a PCP has very important

implications for women, because their doctor's training includes very limited exposure to many important areas in medicine. There are significant gaps in the training of obstetrician-gynecologists that compromise their ability to function effectively as primary care physicians. These deficiencies have been acknowledged by the American College of Obstetrics and Gynecology, which is now sponsoring continuing medical education courses for established physicians in order to retrofit their membership for this new, sought after, expanded role. In addition, many practicing obstetrician-gynecologists have been reticent to assume a significant role in primary care in large part as a result of the recognition that their training and experience has not prepared them for the management of complex medical problems. Recently, residency training programs for obstetrics and gynecology have been modified to include exposure to those subjects in medicine that will permit these specialists to assume the role of a PCP. These initiatives are so new that their results have yet to be demonstrated. However, it is troubling that residents and newly minted obstetrician-gynecologists have been very critical of the primary care training they have been receiving. There has been a very heated debate among more senior obstetrician-gynecologists about the appropriateness of their assuming the role of a primary care provider, although many of their juniors want to take on this responsibility. These younger doctors want to expand their mandate but have been candid in admitting that they do not feel prepared to deliver high-quality general medical care. A very disturbing effect of the new emphasis on primary care in the ob-gyn residency has resulted in short-changing the surgical aspects of the training program. The question being asked, more and more frequently by those involved in the training of ob-gyn residents at academic medical centers, is: Are we doing a disservice to women by producing gynecologic surgeons who many feel are other than superbly trained?

I would recommend that you not select an obstetrician-gynecologist as a primary care physician if you are over forty and have completed child-bearing, since the likelihood of experiencing significant medical problems normally outside of the gynecologists' purview increases with age.

On balance, if you don't have any identified significant illness such as diabetes or high blood pressure, choose your PCP based on the physician's personal competence and the patient-physician chemistry. If you have a serious chronic disease, you should lean toward selecting a board-certified internist as your PCP.

Non-M.D. Primary Care Providers—Keep Your Distance

As a result of new initiatives, you may be surprised to find nonphysician providers such as nurse-midwives, nurse practitioners, or advanced practice nurses and physician assistants providing primary care. Like physicians, each of these groups are licensed and operate under regulations mandated by the division of the state government that supervises health professionals. As a rule, they provide primary health care services to patients under the direction or supervision of a physician. However, in many institutions, nurse practitioners are being given independent hospital admitting privileges and are able to prescribe medications. With the ability of nurses to subspecialize in such fields as pediatrics and gynecology, these nurse practitioners have achieved a functioning status of doctor even at some major academic medical centers.

Regrettably, there are even fewer resources and standards to which patients may turn for information concerning the qualifications of such nonphysician health care providers. Can the average nurse practitioner be better prepared to provide medical care than the average physician? This is not a trick question. I believe the answer is self-evident.

The risk of failing to diagnose a significant problem has been shown to be inversely related to one's training and experience. Certainly no one would seriously suggest that a nurse-midwife or advanced practice nurse would be as skilled in performing a breast or pelvic examination on a menopausal woman as a well-trained, experienced gynecologist.

I am at a loss to understand, given the number of well-trained physicians available to provide the required medical expertise, why anyone would willingly choose a nonphysician as a primary care provider. I would strongly recommend against it. Yet there is a concerted effort on the part of many managed care organizations to promote these non-M.D. providers; I can only surmise that they are motivated by the drive to reduce the costs of care. Since your primary care provider is the first doctor you'd call and the facilitator of your entry into the health care system, you're looking for a relationship that will continue over time.

YOUR PCP—A CRITICAL DECISION

- Your PCP can be a specialist in internal medicine, pediatrics, obstetrics and gynecology, or family practice or a nonphysician nurse practitioner.
- If you want one PCP for the entire family, you should choose a family practitioner.
- If you are over forty or have an ongoing medical problem, a specialist in internal medicine is your best choice.
- Avoid choosing an ob-gyn if you are a woman over forty who has completed child-bearing.

- If encouraged to choose a nonphysician practitioner, just say no!
- In any event, you should pick a PCP with excellent credentials who practices at a convenient location and whom you find communicative, comforting, and convincing.

The third article of the Declaration of Informed Medical Consumer is: "It is imperative that I take an active role in understanding what I want and what I need and finding a qualified person who can fill the role and provide the necessary care."

Choosing Specialists

In many managed care programs, the PCP provides the necessary permission to visit a medical specialist and/or points you to the provider of approved resources, thereby effectively controlling your access to the higher, more sophisticated levels of medical care.

Today, specialist physicians outnumber the generalists. In fact, a substantial number of patients see only specialists for their medical care. Selected specialists often assume the generalist role, particularly when they provide the majority of outpatient care for an individual patient. In the era of managed care, this decision, heretofore in the hands of the physician, may now be under the control of the managed care company.

There are two general classes of specialists. Nonprocedure specialists are physicians consulted for their judgment and opinion about the management of medical problems such as diabetes, cancer, heart disease, or AIDS. The other group of specialists perform procedures and are often referred to as "procedurists." These are surgeons, including orthopedists, urologists, gynecological surgeons, and non-surgical specialists who perform invasive procedures like colonoscopy, angiography, or angioplasty.

What you want and what you need from a specialist physician is very different from that of a primary care doctor. While all medical care requires clinical judgment, any procedure, from something that appears to be simple such as aspiration of fluid from a breast cyst or the thyroid gland, to something as obviously complex as open-heart surgery, demands such physical attributes as manual dexterity, tactile sensitivity, depth perception, hand-eye coordination, and, in some instances, physical strength. Therefore, an entirely different set of issues must be considered when establishing a relationship with a specialist who does procedures. (A detailed discussion of medical procedures appears in Chapter 4.)

Pick-a-Doctor—The Referral Racket

I recently received a telephone call from the editor in chief of a prestigious magazine of scholarly opinion. His call was prompted by concern about a professional colleague and good friend who had just learned that he had prostate cancer. The editor's questions were well focused. He wanted to know my opinion about the two urologists his friend's PCP had recommended. Coincidentally, I had recently had a conversation with the chief of the urology service at a major medical center in New York who had made unsolicited, unfavorable comments about these two doctors. I am clearly not able to judge their qualifications and must rely on professional colleagues whom I judge to be acknowledged experts.

Since it was clear to me that the editor was genuinely

concerned about his friend, and in view of the complexity of the problem and the gaps in his understanding of this friend's condition, I suggested that it would be best if I were to speak with the patient directly. Happy to be unburdened of this responsibility, the editor accepted my offer immediately.

My half-hour conversation with the patient resulted in his deciding to review his options with three different physicians that I recommended—a urologist, a radiation therapist, and a medical oncologist, all of whom I knew had extensive experience in treating prostate cancer.

The most striking thing about these two exchanges is that I had never met either the editor or the patient. The editor's exposure to me was limited to several telephone conversations about an article I had submitted to him for publication. He had, to my knowledge, no rigorous way to evaluate my clinical knowledge with respect to his friend's serious problem, which was clearly not within my area of expertise. The patient himself, who had never met or spoken to me, had no way to evaluate what I was telling him. Yet by the end of our telephone conversation, based solely on what I had told him, he had discarded his original plan of action.

I pointed out to the patient that the surgeons to whom he had been referred by his physician all practiced at the same hospital as his general physician. The patient appreciated immediately the implications of this relationship.

Most referrals made by physicians are based on a mix of factors that rarely include an intensive and often frustrating search for the doctor who would be best for the care of a patient with a specific problem. It is common practice for physicians to refer patients to other doctors on the staff of the hospital to which they admit their patients. While it is true that the referring physician would probably be more familiar with the skills and interests of a colleague than he would of someone with whom he or she does not have professional contact, referrals are a two-way process, and it is common for physicians to maintain a network of physician referrals that are mutually beneficial. This agenda can contaminate the process of patient referrals.

I was struck recently by the fact that women with breast cancer whom I referred to one surgeon were being offered a new surgical approach to evaluate whether the disease had spread beyond the breast. I raised this issue with another surgeon, to whom I also referred patients, who was not employing this strategy. After a lengthy discussion it became clear that the second surgeon was unwilling to even review the data that supported the use of the new technique for staging breast cancer. He made it clear that he intended to continue the more extensive surgical procedure. He admitted that the method he employed was associated with a significant complication that was avoided with the newer approach, but he claimed, "In my hands, that risk is small." I wondered which my patients would choose: an acceptably small chance of having a complication or avoiding it completely with the newer procedure. And of those who had experienced the complication, who would find this doctor's view of its low risk acceptable. He made no claim that the new technique was not as safe or effective. Only after this discussion was it clear to me that, everything else being equal, I should no longer include him among the physicians to whom I referred my patients with breast cancer.

The Search for Quality

Whenever I am faced with the question as to whether a particular patient has received good medical care, I am reminded of Supreme Court Justice Potter Stewart's rejoinder about obscenity. Admitting difficulty in defining it, he declared, "I know it when I see it." That's how I feel about defining high-quality medical care. It isn't easy. Regrettably, there is very little available data to help the consumer choose the better practitioner. In fact, it is just not possible to make a very refined measure of medical quality. You can't expect to differentiate by the inch. In many cases, you can't even discriminate by feet and have to settle for yards. As I pointed out, in very few cases is there a "best." In the vast majority of cases, there are ways to tell the difference between the very good, the good, and the crummy. It is our aim here to make sure you get into the "good' category. It will take some effort on your part to move upstream to the "very good." There are a host of resources for you to research. Each has faults and requires that you maintain a high degree of skepticism about any of their conclusions.

The mystery surrounding medicine and the popularized image of the infallible physician led to an almost unbreakable grip on the profession's control of what are defined as acceptable medical practices. It is only recently that the public has recognized the sorry state of much of health care in the United States, and has attributed this to the arrogance of the medical profession and its insularity and refusal to enter into full and honest discussion with patients.

Astonishingly, until the beginning of this decade, there has been a lack of interest, on the part of academic medicine as well as the state licensing agencies, in quality of care issues. In fact, there was more uniformity of physician skills prior to the admission of large numbers of foreign-trained physicians into the United States. Today, abundant data demonstrates that there are substantial variations in medical practice and treatment of patients with the same condition in different locations. Very slowly, we're starting to see increased interest in evaluating the effects of different treatments.

The National Practitioners Data Bank (NPDB) includes background data on practicing physicians with regard to state licensing agency or hospital disciplinary actions, malpractice suits, or other significant adverse actions of interest to hospitals considering physicians for appointment to their attending staff, as well as such professional groups as peer review organizations, group practices, and managed care organizations. Unfortunately, under current regulations, the NPDB cannot be searched by individuals. There are, however, many efforts under way by a variety of consumer groups to open this resource to the general public.

Although the efforts to create quality measures has thus far generated only very preliminary results, there are today a number of public report cards that rate both doctors and hospitals that are available to patients. *Consumer Reports' Digest, U.S. News & World Report*, and *Newsweek* publish rankings of health plans and hospitals that address patient satisfaction and issues of quality of care. The Agency for Health Care Policy and Research and the Health Care Finance Administration, organizations of the federal government, have major programs to develop, evaluate, and publicize quality measures for health plans and other medical care services. Many of these resources are not currently available to the general public, but these policies are changing rapidly. Today, several states, including New York, Pennsylvania, and Massachusetts, have also taken on this task. The Health Cost Containment Council in Pennsylvania has an on-line listing of data about surgeons who perform coronary bypass. In New York, *www.health.state.ny.us* is a resource with similar data for New Yorkers. These data include death rates adjusted for severity of the disease of the patients included in the doctor's case load, the number of cases the doctor has done, and for each heart surgeon the statistically calculated expected number of deaths. Pacifi-Care Health Systems, *www.pacificare.com,* has a ranking of the more than one hundred doctor groups in California based on a variety of services and patient outcomes. The Pacific Business Group on Health in San Francisco has a similar data base that includes information on more than fifty physician groups in California, Oregon, and Washington, *www.healthscope.org.*

A striking proactive stance has recently been taken by the specialty boards with a move to establish methods of monitoring the quality of their members' practices and programs for remediation of physicians whose activities are judged to be inadequate. Rather than relying primarily on consumer complaints, the boards are investigating methods to evaluate patient outcomes and/or other measurable indices of competency. These initiatives will not meet with the approval or acceptance of most physicians, who have a reflexive distaste for evaluation and audit of their activities. They will not be implemented without a prolonged and protracted debate. And as with the National Practitioners Data Bank, the data that have been collected are not available to the public.

There have been proposals put forward by many state regulatory bodies that would permit publication of information about hospital disciplinary actions with respect to their doctors, arbitration awards, malpractice settlements, and unresolved criminal and civil suits. If you are considering using a physician, you can contact your state licensing agency to see if the doctor has any complaints on file or a record of previous offenses that would affect your decision. While many state disciplinary actions are already in the public domain, we're not yet at the point where such information is uniformly available. To find out whether this information can be obtained, contact the state medical licensing agency. The local county medical society, listed in the telephone directory, will provide you with the address and phone number of the state agency. Initiatives have been taken recently that well may result in such data being available on the internet in all states by the end of 2000.

A caveat! There is evidence that for many physicians there is no correlation between their malpractice history and their competence. Physicians who treat patients with complex illnesses or who use high-risk technologies can end up with more malpractice suits. Consider, for example, the orthopedic surgeon who re-operates on the patient whose first hip replacement procedure has failed, or the cancer specialist who cares for a high number of patients whose disease has relapsed after treatment.

Heart surgery has been the central focus of many of the efforts to create a basis for comparing the results of different cardiac surgeons. Heart surgery is most frequently an elective procedure and is associated with a significant risk of complications and death. There can be as much as a 500 percent difference in the mortality rates among doctors and hospitals. I find it astonishing that the data about this enormous variation in outcomes is rarely considered by patients when selecting a surgeon. It is just foolhardy to find yourself being operated on by a doctor for whom you have not examined and compared the data for that hospital and that doctor with others in your community or region. It is essential for patients to check out these reports from governmental agencies or the news media.

New Ways of Evaluating Doctors

There are currently more than a quarter of a million physicians in the United States who are not board-certified. While most of them are completing their training or finishing the requirements for certification, close to 100,000 physicians describe themselves as specialists even though they have not completed the requisite training or have failed the board examination despite several attempts, or have never even taken the certification exam. You should know if your physician is in this group.

Although certification by one of the American Boards of Medical Specialties was never meant to convey the privilege to practice, it has become and is widely accepted as the standard index of a physician's ability. While certification of an ABMS board is no guarantee of excellence, and lack of certification is not prima facie evidence of lack of competence, the consumer movement has resulted in increasing pressure to more rigorously define the "good" doctor.

There is a new initiative being undertaken by the American Medical Association (AMA) known as the American Medical Accreditation Program (AMAP) that is an attempt to create a standard for physician accreditation. The AMA hopes this program will replace the current patchwork of overlapping assessment systems with a uniform national quality standard for physicians in every form of practice. Their stated goal is to provide consumers with an accessible database of physicians that includes credential verification, physician office assessment, clinical performance evaluation, and patient outcome measures. New Jersey is the first state to officially institute this program in collaboration with state and county medical societies and other local groups. The AMA expects to have this program implemented nationwide by 2002.

At the moment, AMAP has several primary requirements that include graduation from an accredited medical school, an active medical license, and an unrestricted registration with the Drug Enforcement Administration and an absence of disciplinary actions by that regulatory agency. A variety of additional criteria have been established, each of which is associated with a point award. These include completion of a residency program approved by the respective board of the ABMS, certification or recertification by an ABMS board, minimal or no experience with malpractice litigation, no record of adverse actions in the National Practitioner Data Bank, membership in a medical association that subscribes to the AMA's Principles of Medical Ethics, completion of continuing medical education courses, participation in a clinical continuous improvement project, and an office site review. Two additional measures, physicians' performance and patients' outcomes, are to be implemented. To become accredited by the AMAP, a physician needs to accumulate one half of the possible twenty-two points from these supplementary standards. The details about the AMAP and information about specific physicians are available through the AMA in Chicago and its web site, *www.AMA-ASSN.org.*

The AMAP program is bound to be problematic for patients. The standards it has established are minimal, and very few participants in the AMAP program will fail to gain accreditation. Critics claim AMAP will do nothing to guarantee that the public will be better able to evaluate data on individual physicians. My feeling is that while the system is flawed, it will give you ready access to basic information on doctors. This can only help in your decision-making.

Weeding Out Bad Doctors

In 1997, only 3,728 physicians in the United States out of 730,000 were disciplined by their state regulatory agencies as reported by the Federation of State Medical Boards. This number stands in marked contrast to the assertion by the Citizens Health Research Group, a nonprofit consumer agency, that there are at least 10,000 physicians whose activities—including criminal convictions, documented evidence of overprescribing restricted drugs including narcotics, personal alcohol or drug abuse, and sexual misconduct with a patient—would justify their censure or limitation of their practice of medicine. There are striking differences in the rate of serious disciplinary action from one state to another. In Mississippi, almost 12 of every 1,000 doctors faced some serious sanction—a rate that is seven times that in Minnesota. It is difficult to identify the sources of these discrepancies, but clearly state medical licensing authorities are becoming more willing to take away a physician's license as well as to restrict the practice privileges of offending doctors.

A comprehensive list of doctors who have been disciplined by state and federal agencies was recently published. *Questionable Doctors,* by the U.S. patients' advocacy group Public Citizen, details 16,638 physicians in the United States and the more than 34,000 disciplinary actions taken against them. In the newly published volume, 393 doctors are named who have been disciplined for sexual abuse of or sexual misconduct with a patient. Almost 2,000 have been convicted of crimes and 1,309 have been found to be substance abusers. More than 2,300 have been judged guilty of incompetence, negligence, or of providing substandard care. Over 1,500 have been found guilty of wrongly prescribing or oversubscribing drugs. Regardless of the documented offense, fewer

than two thirds of these physicians were required to stop practicing medicine, even temporarily.

As staggering as these numbers are, they represent only the tip of the iceberg. A recently published report on the incidence of the inadvertent laceration of the baby during a cesarean section revealed that no record was made of this injury at the time of delivery in a significant number of the babies included in the study. How many of such injuries were never reported or acknowledged?

Even the National Practitioner Data Bank, which includes the details of any adverse actions taken against a physician, appears to be an incomplete record of documented physician error or incompetence.

Inadequate Doctors, Inadequate Training

American medicine has been dominated by the drive to deliver error-free medical care. Two ominous trends have recently been recognized. The first is that over the past fifteen years, medical students and residents have received progressively less and less exposure to the practical aspects of clinical medicine. This trend is a harbinger of an inevitable deterioration in the level of care that physicians will deliver to their patients. Secondly, it is known among physicians that many of their number do not understand even the most basic day-to-day issues. Many fail to keep abreast of new information, and undertake the care of patients with problems for which they are unqualified by virtue of their training and experience.

It is unrealistic to assume that ability is distributed any differently among physicians than it is among teachers, lawyers, plumbers, or airline pilots. However, the performance of very few physicians is so flawed as to come to the attention of state licensing bodies or result in public

knowledge of their incompetence as a result of the volume of malpractice suits brought against them.

A frightening reflection of the current state of affairs was recently widely publicized. It is a vital task to diagnose important heart problems on the basis of murmurs, clicks, rumbles, whooshes, thumps, rubs, knocks, snaps, and vibrations that occur in literally fractions of a second but can be heard using a stethoscope. In a study of 453 recent medical graduates from thirty-one different primary care residency programs in internal medicine and family practice, it was shown that where scores of 70 to 80 percent were expected and considered acceptable, only 20 percent of the time did these doctors correctly diagnose a significant heart problem that was readily identifiable with just a stethoscope. The authors of this report suggested that this poor performance was most likely due to inadequate training, and recommended that doctors seeking board certification in family practice or internal medicine be required to pass a test in cardiac auscultation. Amazingly, such a practical examination of this basic skill, the use of a stethoscope, is not currently included in the qualification examinations in any of the primary care specialties.

Physicians have always had a difficult time policing their own. With rare exceptions, once students are accepted at medical school, they will graduate unless they choose to withdraw. There is the implicit assumption that the selection process for medical school admission will eliminate those unsuited to the profession. As I've said, this concept is continued through a code of silence that persists throughout medical training and into the years of practice. The reason physicians have so much difficulty evaluating their peers is because they *are* peers; they cannot possibly ignore the cautions "There but for the grace of God . . ." or "Let him who is without blame cast the first stone." Even in the best

GETTING THE RIGHT DOCTOR / 107

of hands following accepted standards of care, it is possible to experience a bad outcome. The real problems are the many cases where the proper attention has not been paid or when egregious deviations from appropriate care are ignored. This is one of the most damaging behaviors of the profession, yet little has been done to correct it. Physicians know that any action to discipline one of their own can have severe consequences, including the ending of a career. As a result, even in the face of repeated errors with serious consequences, there is a quite natural tendency to avoid dealing with problem physicians. Caveat emptor!

Interviewing Your Prospective Doctor

In marked contrast to what is known within the profession, almost every poll reveals that patients believe there is great uniformity in the skills of most physicians and hold their own physicians in high esteem. The majority believe that their doctors are up-to-date with the science of medicine. More than half of the respondents in an American Medical Association poll felt that doctors care about people today as much as they did in the past. However, in these surveys, the three areas of greatest patient dissatisfaction involved the limited information physicians are willing to provide to the patient, the amount of time they are willing to spend in discussion, and the fees they charge for their services.

When one poll asked patients how they chose their physician, 47 percent based their decision on recommendations from friends or family, office location is the primary factor for 27 percent, 24 percent limit their choice to physicians who participate in their health insurance plan, and only 17 percent were primarily concerned with the doctor's qualifications.

Physicians currently spend more than $100 million a year advertising. These promotional activities tend to confuse the decision-making process by affecting the perceptions of the physician's attributes. The existence of this new, now near epidemic of physician PR highlights the lack of relevant and reliable data concerning physician quality. It is a testament to their search for more patients and adds to the complexity of the problem that patients must now resolve. These advertisements should be recognized for what they are: an attempt to bring in business in order to improve the bottom line.

Frequently, I was consulted for a second opinion where the patient made it clear that if I deemed the surgery necessary, I would do the operation, and the fee for surgery could be $5,000. So, many times physicians are required to make decisions that are against their own financial self-interest. I worry about the inherent conflict between this ethical principle and a self-promoting advertising campaign.

> The fourth article of the Declaration of the Informed Medical Consumer is: "I must not be intimidated. I must ask my doctor at least as many questions as I ask my hair dresser or automobile mechanic."

Before you make an appointment with a physician, know the answers to the following questions:

- Are you board-certified?
- When were you certified?
- Where were you trained? What medical school and which residency?
- Where do you admit patients who need to be hospitalized?
- What is your title on the hospital's staff?

Everything being equal, you want to be treated by a board-certified physician who has had some practice experience after completing his or her residency. The doctor trained in a university-based residency has in all likelihood had a greater exposure to unusual or infrequently encountered illnesses. The hospital where the doctor admits his patients should be acceptable (see Chapter 3).

Before you leave the doctor's office at your first visit, you should know the answers to the following questions:

- How frequently have you taken care of patients with my problem who are like me? (The right answer is more than a few.)
- How did they do? (This is the opportunity to learn about the complications that can be expected and what happens when they are encountered.)
- What other doctors do you think will be involved in my care? Tell me about them, their training and experience. (Each of these doctors should go through your critical review.)
- Why did you choose these doctors specifically? (This will allow you to get some insight into how your doctor thinks about these decisions.)

DON'T EVER SELECT A DOCTOR

- From the Yellow Pages
- Based on advertisements
- Without at the very least checking his or her credentials
- Who is unwilling or unable to answer your questions
- Just because a celebrity uses the same doctor
- Just because you saw him on television or heard her on the radio

Office Practices

When I first entered practice, one of my mentors emphatically told me, "Don't ever forget the three most important things to a patient, in order, are: first, accessibility; second, affability; and last, ability." During my years of practice, this point has been repeatedly reinforced by my patients. I am convinced this is because accessibility is easy to determine, affability is subjective, and ability is very difficult to measure. So naturally such factors as office location, office hours, and the friendliness of the office staff and the physician assume great importance in the selection of a physician.

Although I am convinced that these characteristics should be given far less weight than ability, it is critical that patients be able to have reasonable access to their physician and find their doctor willing to listen to them and able to fully discuss their concerns.

If you find that interactions with a specific physician or his or her office staff are problematic but you're satisfied with all the other issues involved in the selection of this physician, it is important that you attempt to discuss it with both the physician and the staff to see if these problems can be resolved.

Personally, I have made it a practice not to recommend any physician with whom I have not worked or have had the opportunity to evaluate his or her clinical judgment and skills. I have not referred patients to surgeons I have not watched operate and seen them cut and sew. Since I am constantly being asked to give an opinion about a physician for whom I do not have this firsthand data, I, too, must fall back on those elements of a doctor's record that are readily ascertainable. In these circumstances, my opinion is couched with many caveats, since it is based on incomplete data and therefore likely to be flawed.

Distribution of Quality

The familiar bell-shaped curve is used to describe characteristics for a variety of things, from the expected life of lightbulbs to the abilities of airline pilots. There are some very good pilots and some very poor ones. The rest, with average skills, are in the middle of the distribution. When we get on an airplane, we hope that the pilot is among the best. The real issue for passengers is will the captain be adequate if there is a problem and the going gets rough. The average pilot will be adequate in most situations. It is for the tough situations that commercial airlines buy added insurance in the form of the second officer, the copilot, who is also qualified to fly the airplane.

The bell curve is a good representation of the skills of doctors, too. Never forget that 50 percent of medical school graduates are in the bottom half of their class, and one in twenty is among the lowest 5 percent. Like airline pilots, most doctors can deal with simple problems. For doctors, the majority of illnesses they will be called on to treat are equivalent to simple airplane takeoffs and landings. In fact, they are even better, since most illnesses will get better regardless of what a doctor does or doesn't do. It's when things are not quite that simple that the selection of a physician is critical. When choosing a doctor, the first question you must ask yourself is, Do I have a simple, straightforward health problem? If the answer to this question is unequivocally yes, you have far greater latitude, and a mistake will be far less costly or potentially damaging than if you have a significant problem.

With a serious illness, the central issue in choosing a physician is that it is not a relationship of equals. When applied to medicine, the consumer paradigm fails to focus on the gross inequality between the patient and the physician in terms of the most vital component of the interaction: specialized technical knowledge. Regardless of how well informed you are about your problem, at many critical junctures decisions will have to be made, and at those times you will have to rely on your physician's judgment.

Because hundreds of lives may be lost at one time, every airline accident is followed by a detailed examination of the facts by governmental agencies. Frequently, the final conclusion of these investigations is that the mishap was attributable to pilot error. *There is no such public review in medicine.* It is because such data are not available that patients' decisions are subjective opinions based on incomplete information.

Medicine shares many similarities with such other high-risk enterprises as flying airplanes, operating nuclear power plants, and race-car driving. The estimated contribution of human factors to accidents in hazardous technologies varies between 30 and 90 percent. In the classification of accidents, active failures are those unsafe acts committed by the point people in the system; in medicine these are usually the surgeon, anesthetist, nurse, radiologist, and pathologist. Latent or delayed failures are those that are derived from higher level flawed decisions or acts that usually involve more than one person. In medicine, the damage done by such latent failures may remain hidden for some time. They often become evident only when they are combined with additional active failures or other latent faults.

At the skill-based level, human performance is the pivotal element in the equation. In addition to fundamental defects in ability, skill-based errors are often attributable to loss of focus. Complex tasks including many medical procedures can become automatic. Skill-based errors are often the result of cutting corners. Much of medicine is based on memory-stored operating principles that are acquired by training and perfected through experience. Mistakes are the result from the misapplication of good operating principles or the application of bad principles. Knowledge-based errors are an attribute of the learner. Rule-based errors are deliberate acts that deviate from accepted standard operating procedures.

As the management of sick patients is more and more a function of the decisions of an increasing number of health care providers, medical outcomes have become very complex events. In this setting, problems can arise and go unnoticed. Even the consequent failure can pass without recognition of its root causes. This is especially true with unexpected or rare events. The relationships between physicians, surgeons, anesthesiologists, nurses, and residents are increasingly more important in the treatment of serious medical problems.

It has been suggested that rather than attending to failures in medicine it would be far more valuable to concentrate on studying excellence. This natural tendency is graphic demonstration of the almost universal desire to avoid the discomfort of confronting one's errors.

But knowledge grows through the recognition and intensive study of error. The tradition in medicine has been to behave as if physicians function without error, and this has led to an environment that is intellectually dishonest. Mistakes are not admitted. Errors are covered up and opportunities for improvement are ignored. The reality of malpractice suits remains the prevailing justification for these behaviors.

Although it is a great error not to admit a mistake, it is

the rare physician or surgeon who openly admits his or her fallibility. In complex settings where outcomes are a function of collective behavior and responsibility, it is often difficult to identify those who are at fault. This has been a major factor in dealing with mistakes, errors, and bad outcomes in medicine as we attempt to simplify explanations to patients and their families. When there is a bad outcome, many times the explanations given to patients emphasize their own culpability while minimizing or denying the physician's role in the process.

Marketing Medicine, or How Not to Choose a Doctor

When one considers how people choose their doctors—from lists of physicians who are members of their managed care plan; referral from other physicians, friends, and relatives; from institutions such as hospitals, medical schools, and professional groups; and even from magazine advertisements—the most important elements in the decision are often ignored.

The "best doctor" lists that appear in a variety of forms and formats are viewed by the informed medical community as fundamentally flawed. Whenever I look at these lists, I am often as surprised by who is included as by those whose names do not appear who I know are superb physicians and have made major contributions to their field. It is especially interesting to find someone included who is no longer in practice, retired, or dead. Once a name is included on such a roster, it is apparently unlikely that it will be removed. While most physicians included in these lists are usually competent, it is clear that many are included simply as a result of their personal relationships with nominating colleagues or their own efforts at self-promotion. Clearly, most physicians would prefer to be included in such lists. There is no doubt that the benefits of inclusion are quickly measured by the increase in new patient visits.

A book has recently been published with an ambitious title that suggests it is a compilation of the best doctors in the New York area. On close inspection, the authors have relied predominantly on professional reputation and claim, albeit vaguely, that their recommendations are based on some undefined research.

When using any such lists, you have no way of knowing which of the "best" are really terrific or of learning the names of those excellent physicians who have not been included. The spreading practice of physicians retaining public relations experts in order to increase their chances of being included in the next "best doctor" list is a reflection of the importance they place on them. You should be aware that these lists are created without the kind of process that *Consumer Reports* uses for evaluating a television set or toaster oven.

In the past, most physicians viewed advertising as unprofessional behavior. Currently, many individual physicians, physician groups, and hospitals spend as much as 10 percent of their annual operating budget on advertising including print and electronic media as well as billboard posters. Marketing consultants advise their doctor clients to get a "good" toll-free number to facilitate patient contact and use a "catchy slogan" to attract new patients.

Physicians retain public relations experts to promote their name to the media in hopes of their being interviewed as an expert on some topic of interest that will be covered in a story in a newspaper or magazine or the subject of a television report. This is a platform for self-promotion that is without cost to the doctor and absent any stigma of being unprofessional.

"Best doctor" lists, advertising, and public relations experts are the insignia of our national infatuation with the marketing tools that have worked so well for selling soap and filling hotel rooms. Why not use them for promoting surgeons and hyping hospitals? Has it occurred to you how many, many millions of dollars are currently being spent by major medical institutions and pharmaceutical companies targeting you directly for services you cannot go out and use or medications that you cannot buy directly?

These marketing tools now include the institutional "referral services" that are operated by managed care organizations, hospitals, medical schools, and clinical departments at medical centers. While there is the appearance that the name you are given when you call the customary 800 number is based on some rigorous data that discriminates one physician in the registry from another, more often than not the name you are given is chosen by a method that attempts to be equitable to the physicians on the list who fulfill the criteria you have specified. For example, if you request a female physician who has an office in a specific area and sees patients on Tuesdays or Fridays, the operator will plug these specifications into the computer and come up with a list of candidates who fill that bill of particulars. If you request a doctor who specializes in psoriasis, you will be given names from among those physicians who have chosen to have themselves listed as having an interest in this disease without regard to any information with respect to their expertise. The important point is that the vast majority of physician referral service recommendations are not based on a rigorous database that certifies that a given doctor has a proven track record in treating a specific disease.

When you call the referral service at a hospital or medical center, you may, in fact, be given the names of the most junior physicians who are just beginning their career. The referral service is a very good way for the chairman of the department to help new staff members build a successful practice. I was one of two physicians who started a practice in gynecology on July 1, 1974, at Columbia Presbyterian Medical Center. The chairman at the time made sure that my name was included in the response to almost every request to the referral service for a gynecologist. I kept meticulous records of the source of all of my new patients and made every effort to maintain excellent relations with the clerks who answered the referral service telephones. These efforts contributed in large part to my consistently seeing a very large number of new patients.

For the majority of problems, you can get by with an average or even slightly below average doctor. It is for the 5 or so percent of problems that require special competency that you need to invest the time and energy required to find someone decent.

Many patients find their physicians through the Yellow Pages. Think about it for a minute. There is absolutely no quality control in any advertising that prohibits or even discourages anyone from making any claim with respect to expertise or experience. In fact, would anyone spend the money to advertise without at least considering embellishing the message? The last thing you need is a surgeon or obstetrician or urologist who uses absolutely uncritical mass marketing. The effects of this kind of thing on a physician's practice, although absolutely independent of any measure of quality, are demonstrated every time his or her name is even mentioned in the press, on radio, or on television. I have had this experience personally when my office was literally flooded with new patient calls after I appeared in a report on the CBS national evening news. A colleague who operated on the New York Yankees pitcher David Cone had the same experience, and I have been told that when radio talk-show host Don Imus made positive comments about his wife's obstetrician and his son's pediatrician, it had a large impact on their patient volume. Every doctor who has lived through this experience knows the benefits of this kind of unprofessional, and therefore uneducated, endorsement.

Personality and Character: The Chemistry of the Doctor-Patient Relationship

There is no correlation between competence and personality. The historic importance of the bedside manner, a crucial attribute for a physician before the advent of the scientific revolution in medicine, heralded by the introduction and widespread use of antibiotics at the end of World War II, has now been relegated to a far less important place in the physician-patient relationship. It is unrealistic to expect that every patient is going to like a given physician or that a physician is going to like every patient. The number of times I have been warned by physicians about patients they are referring to me who they describe as a "pain in the ass" is a testament to the contribution that personality makes to the equation in the physician-patient relationship. This is a two-way street.

This doctor-patient relationship is as subject to personal chemistry as any other interaction. I cannot recall a single lecture in medical school or discussion during my residency about the management or subjugation of my personal likes and dislikes. This subject is only now becoming an integral part of the medical school curriculum. I must admit that there were very few sets of office hours during which I saw only patients whom I liked. Although I had absolutely no way of controlling it, I always hoped that I would see those who were not among my favorites early in the day when I was not too tired to "suffer them gladly."

While your doctor has not had much, if any, training in communicating with patients, it is a good idea for you to decide if his or her manner and your expectations are a good meld. If not, this is a variable that should be included in your equation when choosing a physician. If this is a physician you will be seeing routinely, perhaps for the care of a chronic disease, then give personal chemistry greater weight than if it is a short-term or episodic relationship.

Clearly, you must choose a doctor whom you trust. There will be times when decisions must be made but because of the differences in knowledge base, or other factors, you cannot take an active role in the decision-making process. While at these times it is very important for your physician to understand the mandate you have given him or her, ultimately you must understand that you have placed your life in the doctor's hands. Decisions are best made with your advice and consent but obviously not always with your active participation.

When you quite literally put your life in someone's hands, you want to be sure that he or she will always act in your best interest. This includes telling you when he or she is not up to the task and guiding you to the right person to care for your problem. A physician should not be affected by forces that would deter him or her from following such a path—forces such as his or her own financial self-interest, the parochial interest of an institution or colleague that claims his or her loyalty, or in the economic interest of an insurance company.

You want and deserve a physician whose allegiances are to you. With all the confounding factors that have been discussed here, it is, in fact, a decision that you make that is all about the character of the physician.

After your first visit to a doctor's office, ask yourself the following questions:

Did the doctor willingly answer your questions and provide you with the information you wanted? Remember that, on occasion and for very good reasons, physicians edit their responses to questions—for example, when they don't want to overwhelm you with information or give frightening details at a first meeting. If you are told "Just leave everything to me; I'll take care of it" or some version of this routine, it is appropriate for you to tell the doctor, "I will be anxious unless I know the facts. I believe I am capable of understanding you. I really need to know."

Was there an open discussion of all the treatment options, including the benefits and risks of each one, in order for you be equipped to make an informed decision? You *must* ask about treatment options, and your physician *must* be willing to discuss them with you in detail. There are very few medical problems for which there is just one treatment or approach. For example, there are currently four very different surgical approaches to the repair of a simple, uncomplicated hernia. Each has its pluses and minuses. If the physician is dismissive of you and makes some version of the comment "Don't concern yourself about the details, that's my job," it is a good idea for you to assert yourself by reminding the doctor that it is your problem and that you really need to know your choices in order to make the right decision for yourself.

Do you believe that the physician will be an interested pathfinder and direct you to the right resources and other health care professionals when that is appropriate? The care of patients frequently involves consultation and advice and, at times, the active participation of other medical professionals. You should be assured your doctor recognizes and accepts that.

Did the doctor listen to you? The first lesson the student doctor learns about medical diagnosis is that the patient's history is the vital first step in the process. If the doctor didn't listen to you, the doctor either never learned this axiom or is ignoring it.

Did you feel rushed? If you felt rushed, you probably were. Good medical practice takes time. There really are very few shortcuts that don't significantly compromise quality.

Did the physician appear overworked or exhausted, or overambitious in assuming the ability to treat you regardless of the problem? In the rapidly changing medical care system, it is likely that physicians will feel overworked, tired, and resentful of their loss of autonomy and income. You should be alert to these symptoms of physician burnout, which will affect the quality of the care you receive.

Did you verify that the doctor was well trained, experienced, and, based on data available to you, competent? Remember, this is one of your obligations.

When you left the office, did you know your probable diagnosis and other possibilities? Did the doctor explain the next steps in the process? Were you told the treatment options and were the risks and side effects of each reviewed? Were you told what you could do to reduce the likelihood or severity of side effects? Were you told what would happen if you delayed treatment or did nothing? Did you know when and how the questions that occurred to you after leaving the office would be answered and by whom?

After you review your own feelings and the answers to these questions, you will be well on your way to deciding if this is the right doctor for you.

CHAPTER 3

The Hospital

A big part of the process of choosing a physician should be checking out the hospital where the doctor has what are known as "attending privileges"—that is, where she or he hospitalizes patients. The provider directory you have been given probably includes this information. The reasons you will go to a hospital for care are classified as emergent (it's an emergency; act now!), urgent (take action soon), or elective (schedule it at your convenience). When faced with an emergency, you will have no time to consider the choice of the hospital where you would like to be treated. In these circumstances, where you'll go depends on proximity to the nearest hospital or the choice of the 911 ambulance team. For urgent or elective problems, you have the time to investigate the advantages and disadvantages, strengths and weaknesses of any institution. These aren't trivial distinctions; there are large, and in many instances, growing differences between the best and the worst hospitals.

If It Isn't an Emergency, Don't Go to the ER

If you've ever been to an emergency room, you know that it's the site of periodic episodes of frantic activity punctuated by stretches of comparative quiet. This is where you go if you've suddenly become seriously ill or have sustained a significant injury. Your goal should be to stay out of the ER unless you have a true medical emergency, such as:

- Chest pain; pain radiating into your jaw, down your arm, or into your back; or shortness of breath (If you have acute persistent pain or pressure in the chest, arms, jaw, or throat, call 911.)
- A sudden change in vision, including blurry vision or inability to focus
- Unconsciousness, inability to speak, loss of control of body movements, or unusual numbness of your face, arms, or legs (These could be signs of a stroke or seizure; call 911.)
- A temperature over 104 degrees and/or confusion
- Uncontrolled bleeding from a wound
- Hemorrhage from the mouth, rectum, or vagina
- An apparent drug overdose

Before you ever have to deal with an emergency, you should learn the exact location of the emergency room that is closest to your home and place of business and if they participate in a 911 ambulance response system. If you go to the emergency room for any reason, take a friend or relative who can monitor your care, provide emotional support, and be your advocate or ombudsman with the staff.

Not all ERs are created equal. There are significant differences in the capabilities of emergency room physicians and the resources to which they can turn for help. An ER can be categorized under a variety of state government–controlled definitions and regulations as a trauma center. You should learn which ERs in your area are trauma centers. These will be staffed with physicians specially trained and experienced in critical care specialties and equipped to deal with the most serious emergent conditions.

If you go to an ER that is staffed by physicians who are board-certified in emergency medicine, it isn't realistic for you to expect the same level of care for an eye injury as could be provided by a board-certified ophthalmologist. It is because of this variability in the available skills at a given ER that you should do some research before you need an emergency room about the qualifications of the emergency room staff in the various facilities that you might have to use when faced with an emergency. In addition, you should determine what specialists are readily available if needed. Once the emergency has been resolved, you should request that the appropriate specialist review your condition. If you have broken a bone, you want an orthopedist. If you have a deep cut on your face that requires stitches, you will get a better result if a plastic surgeon sews you up.

If your problem doesn't warrant emergency medical intervention, don't go to the emergency room. The ER staff's top priority is attending to patients with true emergencies. They provide care to the most acutely ill first. If you are not acutely ill, the triage nurse will give you a very low order of priority and you could spend many hours waiting to see the doctor.

If you do go to the ER, be prepared to quickly provide accurate information about your current problem. If you have a complicated medical history, it is a good idea to have it written out in detail in advance and to keep it up to date so you can give it to any doctor. This history should include a list of all prior hospitalizations and surgical procedures, the medicines that you are currently taking with the name, dose, and schedule for taking each one, and any allergies you have to any medication. It is because all this information is already a part of your regular physician's medical records that, if at all possible, you should try to contact him or her first, before you turn to the emergency room for care.

The patient with a true emergent problem has the rights of any patient. For example, a Jehovah's Witness need not accept, and can refuse, a blood transfusion even in the face of a life-threatening hemorrhage. However, if it is an emergency, there is little if any time to have the detailed discussions with the physician that are appropriate in non-life-threatening situations. Once the emergent problem is resolved, all the discretionary issues, including the choice of physician and planned treatment, are ultimately under your control.

Urgent, but Not Emergent, Problems

If you need medical attention for problems after normal physician office hours, there are many local health care centers that provide an alternative resource for nonemergent problems. Many of these are colloquially known as "Doc in a Box" facilities. When you use such an "after hours" center or the emergency room, be sure to take a copy of any records that describe in detail what the doctor or nurse thought and did about your problem to give to your regular physician.

As with all nonemergent conditions, you should determine if the facility you intend to use is a participant in your managed care organization. You can get this information from your managed care company and secure pre-approval, or you will run the risk that your out-of-pocket expenses will not be reimbursed.

Caution: Going to the Hospital May Be Dangerous to Your Health

The hospital is a very complex and, as it turns out, dangerous place for a substantial number of patients. Once you enter its walls, you face the risk of medication errors, negligent nursing care, inappropriate and unnecessary surgery, adverse reactions to blood transfusions and drugs, problems associated with the use of anesthesia, inadequately trained personnel, errors in the interpretation of tests such as X-rays, CAT scans, ultrasounds, and the like by radiologists, and errors in the microscopic examination of biopsy specimens by pathologists. In addition to these risks, the hospital is a reservoir of an enormous variety of infectious diseases for which you are a sitting duck, or a sinking one, since your health was already compromised when you got there.

In 1994, more than 2 million hospitalized patients experienced adverse drug reactions. It was estimated that more than 106,000 died as a result.

Doctors Should Wash Their Hands

The recent increase in the development of antibiotic-resistant strains of bacteria has escalated the risk to patients of developing a deadly infection during hospitalization, especially among postoperative patients. The widely publicized assumption that explains this finding is that physicians are not as vigilant as they have been in the past with regard to the use of sterile technique. From personal experience, I can tell you that I have seen residents on their rounds examine one patient after another without washing their hands. If you see this happening, object—and do so strenuously. It is your vigilance that will be your ultimate protection from exposure to these avoidable risks. How often have you visited a friend in the hospital and seen doctors walking about inside and outside the hospital in surgical scrub suits? The wearing of OR garb outside of the OR is, in fact, absolutely prohibited. Where sterile technique was formerly the catechism in the OR, the disregard of these principles has become epidemic. Such practices as ambulatory patient surgery and hospital admission on the day of surgery, which prohibits the use of antiseptic scrubs and preparation the evening prior to surgery, the increasing reliance and widespread use of prophylactic antibiotics in the pre-, intra-, and postoperative patient have contributed to the undermining of practices that minimized the chance of acquiring a hospital-borne infection.

More generally, it is currently estimated that in the United States, 25 percent of all hospital deaths from pneumonia, heart attacks, and stroke could be prevented by better inpatient hospital care. Five percent of patients get sicker as a result of mishaps that occur in the hospital; 50 percent of these are easily prevented.

Such dangers and their serious implications have not escaped the notice of patients and their families. In a recent Harris opinion poll of fifteen hundred adults, 42 percent reported that they themselves, a relative, or friend had suffered from a medical error in the hospital; 40 percent reported a misdiagnosis that resulted in the wrong treatment; 22 percent received the wrong medication; and an equal number reported a mistake during a procedure. Nearly one third of the respondents had been the victim of more than one significant error. These frightening findings are in line with the experience of any practicing physician.

The official editorial response of the American Medical Association to this data was: "Off with their heads may work with the unscrupulous or the hopelessly inept, but it is a simplistic approach and only partial protection when it is the system itself that may be out to harm patients. . . . Patients may not yet understand the complex issue of protecting them from harm, but . . . there is good reason for hope."

Hospital Outpatient Visits and Inpatient Care

There are more than 300 million outpatient visits to hospitals and more than 30 million Americans spend at least one night in a hospital every year. More than 3 million hospitalized patients undergo invasive procedures. The five most common admitting diagnoses, each accounting for more than a million discharges, are heart disease, obstetrical delivery, cancer, pneumonia, and mental illness.

There are major and significant differences among hospitals in terms of the services that are available and how well they do what they do. Every general hospital offers a variety of services that include general medicine, surgery, pediatrics, and obstetrics and gynecology. Only 20 percent of general hospitals have the facilities for open-heart surgery or the capacity to deliver radiation therapy to cancer patients. An even smaller number of institutions have organ transplant programs.

In addition to recognizing the vast differences among hospitals, you have to accept that in-hospital care is a team process. It is very important that you learn, in advance, whether the team of professionals in a specific hospital has the ability to deal with your particular medical needs. Take out your provider directory, pick up the phone, and find out what departments your hospital has relevant to your health concerns.

Resources for Evaluating Hospitals

Recognizing that it is the complexity of the hospital that is in large measure the cause of individual and cumulative errors, you should be very careful when choosing a hospital. You should first turn to one of the readily available resources that evaluate hospitals.

The Joint Commission on Accreditation of Healthcare Organizations (JCAHO) is the best known and most widely accepted, independent, nonprofit professional organization that conducts assessments of the quality of hospital care and issues certificates of accreditation to hospitals. More than 80 percent of U.S. hospitals elect to participate in the JCAHO program. It is easy to learn the hospital's accreditation status from the hospital's director of quality assurance or directly from the JCAHO service center at (630) 792-5661. JCAHO also has a web site, *www.JCAHO.org,* where detailed information can be readily accessed about hospitals in your region. Reports include the accreditation decision, a summary of the overall evaluation based on their on-site review including performance scores and specific recommendations.

Regrettably, the criteria that lead to JCAHO accreditation are at best very remote measures of clinical outcomes for hospitalized patients. So use the JCAHO report with a grain of salt.

That's the good news. The bad news is that the importance of JCAHO accreditation has led to the practice of hospitals hiding serious medical mistakes. Heretofore, if a significant mishap was reported to the JCAHO, the policy was to immediately conduct an on-site review and place the hospital on an "Accreditation Watch." Under the current JCAHO policy, if an institution voluntarily comes forward within five days of learning of an error that led to the death or serious injury of a patient, the hospital will be given thirty days to conduct a thorough analysis of the mistake's root causes and implement corrective action. Under these conditions, the JCAHO will follow up with a review within six months. The institution's accreditation status would not change and questioners during that time would not be told that an investigation is under way unless they ask about the specific incident. This new strategy is being implemented to remove the current incentives for both physicians and hospitals to hide their mistakes and not reveal the truth.

While there is no doubt that the candid admission of error will result in some lawsuits, the disclosure and evaluation of errors can only lead to an improvement in medical care. Many studies have shown that patients are less likely to sue if they view their doctor and hospital as fundamentally honest. Evidence that a doctor or institution took active steps to conceal a mistake has been shown to cause juries to boost compensatory awards and apply punitive damages. Timely disclosure of errors will allow patients to obtain the necessary treatment, make informed decisions about their care, and receive appropriate compensation.

A reflection of the scarcity of relevant, readily available data for the evaluation of a hospital is the fact that the most widely used, popular hospital survey is the annual hospital guide published by *U.S. News & World Report*. Although the ranking system presented by the magazine is in large part based on subjective data, it represents an important and significant effort to generate a database for patients facing hospitalization. Recently, *U.S. News* has made a substantial effort to include in their measurement system such objective indices as death rates and other variables that reflect a hospital's technological capacity and professional competence.

The importance of the *U.S. News & World Report* ranking is reflected by the use of their published results in the advertising programs of those institutions that have been judged to be among the "Best of the Best." For example, New York University Medical Center invested thousands of dollars for their advertising budget using this slogan until they lost their place in the roster of *U.S. News'* top-ranked hospitals in 1998.

The editorial staff of *U.S. News* modestly claims to provide the "sole source of relevant, rigorously conceived information" for the evaluation of hospitals, while at the same time they admit that ratings are very dependent on "reputational" scores (i.e., subjective). In 1997, eighteen hundred hospitals were included for consideration in the process of ranking the top forty-two hospitals in the United States in seventeen different medical specialties.

The *U.S. News* report is an easy-to-use resource that will be helpful to you if your problem falls within one of the medical specialties included in its survey. I have been impressed by their efforts and believe that as a rule, institutions that have ranked high in one or more of the fields included in their rankings are very likely to be better-than-average providers of care in other related areas of medicine.

As difficult as it is to evaluate the quality of care provided by a physician, the complexity of this process is many orders of magnitude more difficult when the object is a hospital. This complexity is most usually highlighted by the differences between institutions with respect to what is called their "patient profile"—the severity of illness of the patients they treat. In other words, does a hospital have a higher mortality rate because it treats sicker patients who are more likely to die, or because it provides substandard care? Every reasonable study has concluded that severity of patients' illness alone doesn't explain the observed differences among hospitals. But even though we admit that the methods that are available to ascertain important differences among hospitals are flawed, they are the best we have at present, and their use, in the market-driven, highly competitive health care environment, appears to stimulate efforts at quality improvement. As report cards naming individual hospitals appear in morning newspapers and on the evening television news, the responses of those institutions that have received poor grades have been swift and public. In fact, these public reports have been associated with marked changes in the routine practices in many hospitals.

A graphic demonstration of these differences was shown in a California study of patients who have had heart attacks. It led to the inevitable conclusion that all hospitals in that state are not equal. The differences among them are large, with thirty-five out of four hundred hospitals having fewer than the expected number of heart attack deaths and thirty-one facilities having a worse-than-expected record. These results were adjusted to reflect that some hospitals treated sicker patients.

Polls indicate that although there are available data concerning meaningful differences among hospitals, in the majority of cases, the criteria consumers use to define the quality of their hospital are the amenities, food, cleanliness in the hospital, and ease of access or convenient parking. Their second level of concern is that their expectations are met. The third level is that they want to be included in the decision-making process with regard to their treatment options. It turns out that patients are very often satisfied with care that is not high quality and not infrequently dissatisfied even when they have received very high quality care. I need hardly note that I think the evaluation of any hospital should be based on far more rigorous measures of quality care.

The differences among the bases upon which patients and professionals evaluate the quality of medical care are not surprising in view of the continuing and often heated controversy among the professionals about how to measure that quality. While you the patient may be academically interested in the fact that the proper procedures are followed, what you really care about is your own case. You should focus like a laser beam on what happens to you as a result of the treatment you receive. Do you get better? Are you cured? Everything else is little more than window dressing, an amenity, compared to this central issue.

The Performance Measurement Coordinating Council (PMCC) was established by three organizations—the American Medical Accreditation Program (AMAP), the National Committee for Quality Assurance (NCQA), and the Joint Commission (JCAHO)—to develop a common system for evaluating health care at every level. This group intends to focus its attention on providing information on performance to health care purchasers, providers, and consumers. This new initiative of these organizations has as yet no track record but may well be a useful resource for you in the not-too-distant future.

Types of Hospitals

There are a variety of different groups of hospitals in the United States. One classification is based on financial or funding structures. There are voluntary or nonprofit hospitals, some of which are affiliated with religious organizations or universities. There are hospitals that are for-profit institutions that are either privately or publicly owned and may be part of large corporations such as Columbia HCA. Then there are government hospitals operated by the Veterans Administration as well as municipal, county, and state governments.

Teaching and Nonteaching Hospitals

Another and very important division of hospitals is between teaching and nonteaching institutions. As a rule, the usually smaller, nonteaching hospitals are often friendlier, more hospitable places. However, I would use these hospitals only for the treatment of simple, uncomplicated problems such as normal, routine obstetrical care or minor elective surgical procedures. Don't go to one for the treatment of unusual or serious diseases such as cancer or heart disease. Let me explain.

Teaching hospitals are generally larger and more impersonal institutions. They have training programs for physicians in a variety of fields. This is a very important distinction from your point of view since a teaching institution by definition is involved with highly sophisticated technologies in those areas in which they provide specialty training.

At teaching hospitals, the house staff, doctors-in-training, provide twenty-four-hour-a-day physician services and manage patient care under the guidance and supervision of a staff of fully trained attending physicians. If the hospital is affiliated with a medical school, its attending physicians are members of the medical school faculty.

Teaching hospitals have been the target of a litany of familiar and appropriate complaints. They are often large and impersonal. The house staff are often transients who have no time to develop a caring relationship with patients.

These institutions, however, have a greater concentration of clinical expertise and technological excellence. Among the agencies that attempt to measure the quality of hospital care, such as the National Opinion Research Center at the University of Chicago, teaching hospitals regularly are at the top of the list.

Comparing one type of hospital with another in an attempt to measure differences in the quality of care is an elusive goal. Where rigorous attempts have been made to determine if meaningful differences do exist, it appears that patients with hip fracture, heart failure, or stroke who are treated in teaching hospitals have lower mortality rates. It is interesting that nonteaching hospitals score better on measures of nursing care. When one focuses on patients' perceptions, the issues of greatest concern are whether they were given adequate information, whether their pain and discomfort was adequately treated, whether care was coordinated, whether there was continuity of care, and whether their families were involved and considered in the process. These are very different measures than the structure, process, and outcome variables that are included in the most widely read reports on the quality of hospitals.

GO TO A TEACHING HOSPITAL

- If you have a serious illness like cancer, heart disease, stroke, or a life-threatening disease
- If you have a complicated problem like diabetes, rheumatoid arthritis, multiple sclerosis, or high-risk pregnancy
- If you require high-tech care such as sophisticated scanning techniques, the use of new technologies like the gamma knife, the skills and experience of highly specialized physicians
- If you have a choice

Although you may like the geniality and proximity of your local nonteaching community hospital, the quality of care there is usually not of the standard in teaching institutions. Without discounting the importance and comfort to the patient of ready accessibility to family and friends, there really is no legitimate question that the most critical part of the equation for patients who require hospitalization should be high-quality medical care; you should never sacrifice this for either logistical or social reasons.

GO TO A NONTEACHING HOSPITAL

- If you have a simple problem that requires hospitalization, such as normal, uncomplicated obstetrical care, an appendectomy, treatment for uncomplicated problems like pneumonia
- If there is no conventional teaching hospital

There is a practice in teaching hospitals that has recently contributed to a major increase in the cost of care at these institutions. This is commonly known as the faculty practice plan tax, which represents a tithe that the teaching faculty pay to the administration of the hospital, which is in the range of 10 percent of the physician's gross practice income. This is a significant tax and generates a substantial amount of money for the institution while at the same time adding to the cost of care. More than $200 million of revenue were generated for the institution by the taxes levied on medical faculty practice plans at Columbia University in 1996 and 1997. This is a common practice at academic medical centers.

These taxes contribute to making major teaching hospitals the most expensive of inpatient facilities and, as a result, unattractive to managed care companies. However, there is a growing body of data that demonstrates their relative quality and efficiency. A major study completed in 1997 demonstrated that, after adjusting for all controllable variables among the institutions being compared, there was a significantly lower mortality rate for specific diagnoses and length of stay in major teaching hospitals as contrasted with minor teaching and nonteaching hospitals. More specifically, a number of studies have provided consistent and dramatic evidence of the enormous advantage for patients with cancer who are treated in these major centers. The outcome for patients who undergo complex surgery for a variety of cancers has been shown to be best for patients who are cared for in hospitals that treat a large volume of patients with these diseases. Higher volume centers had a dramatically lower postsurgical mortality rate. Studies have also shown that the concentration of the care of children with cancer in a relatively few centers has been one of the most significant factors that contributed to the major progress in this field during the last twenty-five years. This has also been dramatically demonstrated in the survival rates of patients who undergo bone marrow transplant, with the lowest mortality noted in those treated at the highest volume centers. While only a few technically complex procedures have been studied, it is not unreasonable to infer that centers that do a high volume of other complicated surgical procedures associated with intensive and extensive postoperative care as well as operative technical skills of a high order do better than those who do a low volume.

Another study with similar conclusions that was carried out in New York State showed that the volume of coronary angioplasties performed in the hospital and the number performed per cardiologist were inversely related to hospital mortality. Quite simply: The more operations the doctor did, the lower the death rate. Moreover, coronary artery by-pass surgery was done less frequently in these high-volume institutions as a result of an emergent complication of the angioplasty. As with all such relevant information, the best way of learning exactly what the physician and the hospital have done is to ask specific questions. How many of the procedures do you do? What is the mortality rate? Relapse rate? Rate of postoperative complications?

Special Mission Hospitals

Professor Regina Herzlinger of the Harvard Business School, following a corporate model of big business, has proposed that hospitals be organized as "focused factories" designed to deliver health care services that are optimally packaged from the consumer's point of view. In the era of managed care, she suggests that such focused organizations will have financial incentives to invest in patient self-care programs and in the best diagnostic and monitoring systems because this will reduce their exposure to the high cost of caring for preventable problems. At present, this is a theory with some influential proponents but, at this point, little supporting hard data.

The current political environment has made it difficult for managed care to implement many reasonable cost-cutting efficiencies. The variety of legislative initiatives written to prohibit the limitation of in-hospital stay for maternity care for new mothers to twenty-four hours is an example of this problem. Without dealing with the many reasonable approaches to this issue, these laws mandate an extra day in the hospital for the 2 million women who will have uncomplicated vaginal deliveries of normal babies. This could translate into almost 2 million extra hospital days annually. Increasing governmental regulations that are driven by consumer dissatisfaction will result in making it increasingly more difficult for managed care organizations to compete as cost-effective organizations. Even when reasonable medical judgment would justify instituting changes that would reduce medical expenses, political considerations will control the process. This will impede almost any change that is motivated by the goal of reducing medical care costs by managed care organizations.

At a time when changing medical practices and minimally invasive surgical technologies (Band-Aid surgery) are reducing the in-hospital length of stay, the cost of maintaining the elaborate physical plant of state-of-the-art, high-tech hospitals is rapidly becoming prohibitive. The specialized, mission-dedicated hospital is, if for no other reason, the answer on purely fiscal grounds. In this proposed business model, chains of mission-focused institutions, each dedicated to do what it does best, will replace traditional hospitals.

Professor Herzlinger likens these facilities, each treating a specific medical problem, to single-specialty retailers like Staples, the office supply company, and Home Depot, the full-service hardware store, which focus on one niche and are able to do a high volume of business with lower operating costs. As a result of horizontal integration, there will be economies of scale in addition to a base from which the best practices will be developed and replicated among each of the institutions of a given class.

As Professor Herzlinger has pointed out, patients with chronic diseases are more likely to turn to alternative medicine because traditional medicine does not provide them with solutions to their problems. They do this even though it is often far more costly for them, since the services of alternative providers are not necessarily covered or only fractionally covered by most insurance plans. She has suggested that for this reason the first focused health care factories should be for patients with chronic diseases staffed by providers from many different specialties. Such institutions would focus on caring for their customers' chronic diseases and other associated ailments. In an aging population, where more and more of us will live with chronic diseases, this is an idea with a natural and growing customer base.

We already have currently operational "focused factories" dedicated to heart disease; cancer; medical specialties such as pediatrics in hospitals for babies, infants, and children; orthopedics; and ophthalmology. A current financial analysis of this class of institutions suggests that because of their single focus they can achieve efficiencies that allow them to deliver care in the most cost-effective manner. As a result of these economies, they are often the favored providers of managed care programs.

For you, there is good news and bad news about these highly focused institutions. While they are usually on the cutting edge of the management of the problems of central interest to them—and in the age of super-specialization this can be a distinct advantage—their singularity of purpose may result in a relatively low level of competence in dealing with problems outside their special focus.

GO TO A SPECIAL-MISSION HOSPITAL

- If you have the disease they specialize in treating
- If one is conveniently located, and affiliated with a teaching hospital
- If your doctor can participate in your care

An additional caution for the patient is that such prestigious disease-specific institutions as Memorial Sloan-Kettering in New York City and M. D. Anderson in Houston,

Texas, are primarily research centers. The vast majority of their patients are enrolled into what are commonly known as protocol studies in which a patient is assigned a given treatment by a random process. This kind of clinical testing is the only reliable way to determine how effective a treatment is relative to other options. This practice may not be one with which you are instantly comfortable. In many settings, this is the only way that decisions are made with regard to the choice of treatment. You should discuss with your doctor whether or not this is the procedure that is being used prior to initiating any treatment. You are free, without prejudice, to refuse to enroll in any clinical trial.

There is no question that the aspects of specialization, including the training of the doctors, patient caseload, and the formation of multidisciplinary teams confer significant advantages for patients with malignant diseases as breast cancer, ovarian cancer, colon cancer, lymphomas, and leukemia, as well as conditions that require organ transplantation and other complex surgical procedures. Many studies have shown that treatment in cancer centers has many measurable benefits including helping you live longer.

For-Profit versus Not-for-Profit Hospitals

The word *hospital* was originally defined as a charitable institution for the infirm, needy, aged, or young to provide medical care without limitation with regard to the ability to pay. Historically, the hospital was a not-for-profit institution that, in fact, had a significant societal role. There are some concerns about the introduction of the profit motive into the operation of hospitals.

Clearly, a public corporation with an obligation to its stockholder owners has a very limited ability to care for those who cannot pay the bill. For-profit hospitals have a set of operating principles that inevitably affect decisions about the care they provide. The imposition of the corporate profit motive between the doctor and the patient clearly has the potential of imposing restrictions of choice that are not present in the not-for-profit environment. I am less concerned when the for-profit institution is involved in the delivery of such services as cosmetic surgery that is not customarily covered by medical insurance.

The Cost of Hospital Care: Who Pays for What— Always Check Your Bill

Since the end of World War II, the majority of Americans have given little attention to the cost of their inpatient hospital care, since it was customarily paid by third-party health insurers. Even with the advent of managed care, patients continue to delegate the issue of the cost of care to their insurance company.

However, more and more medical insurance policies have a large deductible component or co-pay. This is an important issue for anyone who is directly responsible for any portion of the hospital bill. You must review every item and charge included on every invoice from the hospital.

There is a large variance among hospitals with regard to administrative costs from approximately 24 percent for private not-for-profit hospitals to 34 percent in for-profit hospitals; the most expensive medical facilities are academic medical centers. In addition to this significant differential in administrative costs, the overall costs for care in for-profit hospitals are substantially higher than at not-for-profit institutions. If you are required to pay for any portion of your hospital care, this difference can be very important and personally costly. There have been many studies published that have shown striking differences in the charges between hospitals for comparable services such as a total knee replacement.

Today, the CEO of every hospital, for profit or not, pays strict attention to their market share. In the current environment, when your medical condition permits, you should comparison shop for medical care among equivalent institutions.

The rise of managed care and cutthroat competition have led hospitals to enter into negotiations with insurance carriers for almost every charge they levy for the services they provide. We all know that the person sitting next to us on an airplane probably didn't pay the same amount for his or her ticket as we did. It is no different in the hospital today. For every service provided—chest X-ray, blood test, Pap smear—the charges that a hospital levies are negotiable.

You should view the hospital in no small part as a hotel with a special mission. Just as hotels will voluntarily upgrade guests when they check in, some patients are put in private rooms at no additional cost to them. While you should not discount the potential advantages of having company while confined in a hospital, sharing a room has obvious risks. Ask about the availability of a private room when you are being admitted to a hospital. If you are told that there is a premium over and above your insurance coverage, often this rate can be negotiated. In many hospitals, there are different grades of private rooms. The cost of these varies with current occupancy rates. If you are interested, you should discuss this with the admitting office personnel. It is almost a certainty that after you are discharged from a hospital, you will receive a letter from the fund-raising office asking for a donation. Even if you will never be a substantial benefactor, they want to cultivate your feelings of generosity. Putting you in an otherwise empty private room is a very good strategy and the hospital administration knows it.

There has been some question about the hospital charges for such things as aspirin and Tylenol. If these are not covered by your insurance and you are paying for these out-of-pocket, it is appropriate to bring your own supply to the hospital. You may be asked to turn them over to the nursing staff to ensure that you do not, in error, take the wrong pill or too much medication, which could cause a problem at a time when the institution is responsible for you.

Remember, there is a big difference between what a hospital charges and what they are paid by different insurance carriers, and if you are responsible for some portion of that bill, that difference is going to affect your out-of-pocket expenses. If you are personally responsible for costs associated with your care—for example, if you are to have a procedure such as a tubal ligation that is not a covered service under your health policy—you should learn what the hospital charges under the contracts it has with managed care companies. This charge should provide the base for your negotiation of the bill you will receive for these services.

In this regard, you should ask every physician you see if their services are a part of the hospital routine—that is, covered by your inpatient insurance contract. This is true for all resident or house staff doctors. Do you really want to pay for someone whose role in your care consists of "just dropping by to see how you're doing"? If your doctor has requested a consultation with a gynecologist or cardiologist, you will be responsible for the payment of the fees associated with this care. Be sure that you know who your doctor has arranged for you to see and why. It is also appropriate to ask consultants about their fees and determine if they are participating physicians with your plan. An example of the complexity of the system is demonstrated by the case of the mother of a three-year-old who did not want to change her child's pediatrician when her husband's employer changed insurance plans. They decided to pay for those visits, which were not covered at all out-of-pocket. The child was referred to a specialist for evaluation as a result of recurrent inner ear infections. They were horrified to learn that even though the specialist was a participant in their managed care plan, his $500 fee was not covered by the plan since the referral was from a nonparticipating PCP.

In order to effectively reconcile your hospital bill, it is vital that you know exactly what was done, every test that was conducted, and every medication that you were given during the period of your hospitalization. In addition to the benefit of being able to validate all the charges that are paid by your insurance carrier as well as those for which you are responsible, this information gives you the opportunity to monitor what is happening and have a record of what is being done. This vigilance has the added benefit of reducing the likelihood of your being involved in some untoward event, like being given the wrong test or medication. Bring to the hospital the name, dose, and schedule of administration for every medication your physician has ordered for you. Keep this written record on hand and update it each day so you can verify that every pill and injection you're given has, in fact, been ordered by your doctor. In addition, since you will be subject to such errors as being given the wrong diet or having the wrong X-ray, you should discuss all the specific details of your care with your physician every day. This will decrease the likelihood that you will be subject to an untoward error in your treatment.

You need not be concerned about offending your physician when you ask for this information. Every practicing doctor who has cared for hospitalized patients is well aware that he or she is dependent on a veritable army of nurses, aides, orderlies, technicians, transporters, and dieticians, as well as other physician colleagues. Each of us knows that mistakes can and inevitably will be made in the care of hospitalized patients. Some will get the wrong drug. Some will be given the wrong diet. Some will have the wrong X-ray. Some will not get the correct blood test. In fact, we know that regardless of our personal level of vigilance, these errors are happening with increasing frequency and very often with serious consequences.

In many instances you will not be able to oversee these details, and for this reason, whenever possible, you should have a strong-willed healthy friend or assertive relative to act as your ombudsman, one who will not be easily intimidated in the normally intimidating hospital setting.

When you uncover an apparent discrepancy in a hospital bill, you should raise the issue with the hospital billing department in writing. If you do not receive an adequate explanation for the overcharge, you should address a letter to the chief financial officer of the hospital, including a copy of all supporting documents and your previous letter. If this letter goes unanswered or the response is unacceptable, you should address a letter to the president of the hospital and the chairman of the board of trustees.

If you have made every effort to reconcile the charges that have been included in your bill and have not been able to resolve a meaningful difference, you may want to retain the services of a member of one of the group of consultants called claims adjusters, medical claims consultants, or medical claims assistants. For an established hourly fee, these people will undertake to represent you in resolving a contested claim with a health insurance company, doctor, or hospital. It is clear that the disputed amount of a claim should be at least $1,000 to justify the expense of turning to such a consultant service. In any event, this resource will be substantially cheaper than retaining a lawyer.

Finding a claims practitioner isn't easy. Licensing requirements for these individuals vary widely from state to state. The American Health Information Association in Chicago is a trade group of claims processors. Their address is 919 Michigan Avenue, Chicago, IL 60611. The telephone number is (312) 787-1540. (There is no website at this writing.) This organization requires that these claims processors have completed at least two years of college or have three to five years of experience in addition to passing an examination.

In the Medical Marketplace, a Bargain May Not Be a Bargain

Many studies have shown striking differences in the charges between hospitals for comparable services such as total knee replacement. It is important to examine some of the factors that underlie these differences.

You may not always be able to measure or identify the differences in what may appear to be equivalent procedures. For example, an orthopedic surgeon was recently told by the director of his department that the artificial prosthesis he was using in his patients was much more expensive than other alternatives. The surgeon was angry, since the director acknowledged that the less expensive device was also less durable and more likely to fail after a fixed time interval than the more costly one. When such an implanted prosthesis fails, the patient requires a second surgical procedure that is technically more difficult and is associated with a greater risk of complications than when the original implant was placed. The argument was made that the less expensive device should be used in older patients with a relatively short life expectancy, since it was unlikely that they would outlive its durable life. At the end of their review of this matter, the director of the service pointed out that if they could not come to an agreement because of limitations on the budget, it would become necessary to limit the total number of implant surgical procedures the surgeon could do. It was not necessary to point out the impact of such a limitation to the surgeon, whose income is dependent on the fees generated by the operations he performed.

This is just one example of the complexity of shopping for hospital services, but to be forewarned is to be forearmed. It is an illustration of the level of detail that requires your attention. It is no different from when you hire someone to redo the roof on your home or when you shop for replacement tires for your automobile. Asphalt roofing tiles are much less expensive than cedar wood shingles, and a steel-belted radial tire will have a longer life than other alternatives. Which is right for you? It is not possible for you to appreciate and evaluate all the technical details of a procedure. It is not unreasonable for you to expect that your doctor has this knowledge. It is essential that you discuss all the details of your care with your doctor. The answers to your leading questions—Why is he or she using a specific approach or procedure? What other options has he or she considered? Are the risks and benefits of each comparable?—will provide you with firmer ground on which to base your decision.

As a result of the enormous activities of the consumer movement, most of us have become careful shoppers. We walk up and down supermarket aisles comparing per-unit costs and make choices about everything from soup to nuts.

We are usually curious about the oil that is going to be used when our car is serviced. You wouldn't think about buying an automobile without discussing with the salesman your choices and the costs of all the extras. It is foolhardy to ignore the same operating principles when buying your medical care.

When using a provider who is a participant in your managed care program, your financial exposure is limited to the contractual copayment. While it is not out of the question that your physician may consider reducing that charge, you should recognize that for the most part the fee schedule for managed care enrollees represents a substantial discounting of the physician's normal fees. However, when you choose an out-of-network provider who has quoted his or her customary fee for services, it is not unreasonable to ask if the fee paid by your insurance carrier would be acceptable. While the physician's standard fee may well be double or triple that reimbursed by the managed care company, I can assure you that many physicians will be receptive to this proposal.

This same strategy can be used in dealing with the hospital. You should be aware that under their contracts with the various managed care companies, hospitals have significantly different charges for the provision of identical services. If you are enrolled in a plan that limits your choice of hospital but has an out-of-network payment schedule, and you would prefer to go to a nonparticipating hospital, you should discuss with that hospital's finance officer whether they would be willing to accept this as payment in full. Again, while that amount may differ significantly from what they will quote as their charge, you should understand that, today, "standard" rates are a fiction.

The Hospital Team

From the moment you enter the hospital, your care is provided by a team, and the captain of the team is your physician. The others on the team are usually new faces.

THE MEDICAL HIERARCHY IN TEACHING HOSPITALS

Consultant specialist
Attending physician
Clinical fellow
Chief resident
Senior resident
Junior resident
Intern
Medical student

When you are in a teaching hospital, it is useful to have this list nearby. You should know the rank of everyone involved in your care. Remember, your attending physician is the doctor of record and ultimately the one responsible for your care. Everyone else reports to him or her. Services provided by everyone below that rank are provided without any cost to you.

If you have a question about anything that is being done, you should raise it. If the response is not satisfactory, you should politely ask to see the next higher ranking house officer. If an answer doesn't make sense to you, it may be because it doesn't make sense.

Anyone who has ever been a hospital patient will confirm that within minutes of admission it is made clear that the institutional system is designed to annihilate every vestige of your sovereignty and self-esteem as a mature, self-assured, thinking adult. Standard hospital operating procedures make it difficult for any patient to maintain any sense of autonomy. Soon after being admitted, you are stripped of your clothing, belongings, and freedom of movement. Often you are given medications that can affect your ability to think or speak. You find yourself isolated and almost helpless and in an environment where "good patients" are docile, uncomplaining, stoic, unquestioning, undemanding, and do not take up much of the valuable time of the doctor or the hospital staff.

It is, in fact, the "difficult" patient, the one who is communicative, alert, active, and strong-willed, who does best in the hospital. It is important for you to do everything possible to retain the insignia of a mature adult in charge of his or her fate. Such seemingly trivial things as wearing your own pajamas and robe make a statement to the staff, who tend to think of their patients as just anonymous transients passing through. It will not escape your notice that they have a very proprietary view of "their domain." So although at times this is difficult to do when you meet resistance from some members of the staff, for your own mental health hold the line.

In dealing with any such hierarchical pecking order, you must be sensitive to the feelings and the implicit assault on the ego of anyone whose qualifications or authority you question or challenge. Phrase your questions diplomatically.

In the final analysis, however, you should never forget it is your own physician who has the ultimate authority over your care and who you are paying for all this service. So if you have any hesitancy about undertaking what could become a difficult or uncomfortable interaction, it is entirely appropriate for you to turn any possibly contentious matter over to your own doctor. In my experience, the most effective and efficient way for any of my patients to resolve any issue was to bring it directly to me. In all candor, these were not tasks that I welcomed, but of the two of us, I knew that I was far better prepared to deal with such problems.

THE NURSING HIERARCHY IN THE HOSPITAL

Nurse clinician
Nursing supervisor
Head nurse
Registered nurse
Licensed practical nurse
Practical nurse
Nurse's aide
Orderly

You should make every effort to ensure that the nurses are your allies. It is helpful if you are cheerful, friendly, co-operative, and considerate of them. I recognize that this is no small task when you are sick and feeling crummy. How-ever, since you are dependent upon them, it is vital that you make every attempt to avoid antagonizing them and maintain good relationships with all members of the hospi-tal staff. Remember, it's the nurses who will bring you your medication when you are in pain. The aides will bring you food when you are hungry, an extra blanket when you are cold, walk you to the toilet when you need help, and change your bedding when you have a soiled sheet.

Be sure that you know who is touching you: name, rank, and serial number. And when you are attempting to prove that your challenged autonomy is alive and well, if you feel yourself wavering, it may help you to remember that you are paying for all this!

If things are not what you believe they should be,

ask why. The diplomatic approach to a problem is the best strategy. Your questions should be addressed to the most readily available professional. If you are not satisfied after discussing your concerns with the staff immediately involved in your daily care, you should not hesitate to bring these issues to the attention of your physician. In addition, many hospitals have instituted a Patient Ombudsman program to help you resolve any problems. In every case, you should never forget you have the right to refuse any treatment. And that is exactly what you should do until your questions are answered to your satisfaction.

Your Rights in the Hospital

Every JCAHO-accredited hospital has a Patient's Bill of Rights available for your review. A prominent component of this document is the guarantee that while you are hospitalized, you will be fully informed about all aspects of your treatment.

For many of the procedures that you will undergo as an inpatient, you will be required to sign a consent form. You cannot give an informed consent without knowing exactly what is being done.

Your medical record is a private document and information in it will be confidential. You have the right to read your medical record without charge and to obtain a copy for a reasonable fee.

The Patient's Bill of Rights certifies that you will be provided with a written discharge plan. Its provisions give you the right to refuse to take part in research or to be examined or treated by medical students or doctors in training.

Hospital-Based Doctors

The Hospitalists

In the hospital, you will be cared for by many physicians who are hospital employees. These physicians are commonly referred to as "hospitalists." At present, there is no specialty board that awards certification to hospitalists. Collectively, they will be involved in many important decisions regarding your care.

The hospitalist program has been motivated in large measure by fiscal concerns. Groups involved in paying for medical care want to be sure that such care is delivered as cost-effectively as possible. Hospitalists are expected to balance quality and cost considerations, and are therefore on the front line of those who actually "manage care." This is at the very least a potential for conflict of interest and will require vigilance of a disinterested ombudsman to prevent a compromise of quality. In many institutions, ombudsmen have already proven their worth as agents of both cost and quality control.

Using the National Health Service in England as the model for the delivery of care to hospitalized patients, many hospitals argue that separating inpatient from outpatient care results in the more efficient use of physicians and higher-quality care. You must recognize that the high level of rapidly changing technology that is now routinely employed in the care of hospitalized patients demands a level of expertise that is difficult to achieve and maintain unless the doctors spend the majority of their time caring for the hospitalized sick. So hospitals focus on the delivery of inpatient care, while physicians who provide outpatient care focus on caring for those with less acute or chronic illnesses in their office practices.

Currently, most hospitalists have been trained in general

internal medicine, and some have had more extensive training. A training program designed for physicians who want to
specialize in the care of hospital patients has been initiated
at the University of California in San Francisco. While hospitalists are currently in place in the departments of internal
medicine of many hospitals, the movement is being extended to other major specialties, including pediatrics, obstetrics and gynecology, and surgery. Although there are as
yet no data that would permit the rigorous evaluation of the
effects of this program, it is very likely that if you are hospitalized in the future, a hospitalist will be involved in your
care. If you have questions when you find yourself being
cared for by a hospitalist, you should take an active role to
ensure that your physician remains a player in the process.

Many managed care plans have already embraced this
model of inpatient care as a result of the obvious efficiencies
of the utilization of physician time, the resultant increase in
professional productivity, and cost-effectiveness. I am suspi-
cious that a result of hospitalist programs may well be a loss
of continuity of care. However, it is wise to recognize that
your physician has probably signed on to this program and
appreciates the input of specialists who are focused on the
care of acutely ill hospitalized patients.

This group of physicians has recently formed their own
advocacy group, the National Association of Inpatient Physicians. It is not unlikely that organized labor will attempt to
unionize this group of physicians in the near future.

Intensivists

The physicians known as "intensivists," who staff the
hospital intensive care units, are the prototypic hospitalists.
Critical care medicine, the specialty of physicians who are

responsible for the care of patients in the hospital's intensive care units, has been in existence for more than fifteen years. The critical importance of their role has been demonstrated in a study that showed that where such intensivist expertise was not available, one serious error was committed every two days per patient in the ICU. ICU patients are not in a position to take an active role in overseeing their care and are entirely at the mercy of the ICU staff. They are totally dependent on their personal physician, family, and friends to provide what oversight they can of this high-tech care.

Anesthesiologists

The one-word motto of the American Society of Anesthesiologists is "Vigilance." Considering that when they administer general anesthesia, the patient is unconscious, frequently paralyzed, and the drugs that are being used can affect all of the body's vital functions, it is a situation fraught with hazard. The danger to heart, lungs, brain, and life itself from anesthesia cannot be overstated. Complications— including death—are more common than most physicians believe. The risks associated with anesthesia are underscored by the fact that it is implicated in the deaths of many of the more than 2 million healthy women undergoing a normal obstetrical delivery each year. Inexperience and error are the culprits.

This is not surprising in view of the complex issues that are involved in administering anesthesia, which involves the use of different pharmacologically active agents that have profound depressant effects on the central nervous system as well as widespread potential adverse effects on the heart, liver, lungs, and kidneys. Deaths attributable to anesthesia can occur because of a preoperative omission or error. During operations, errors in anesthesia resulting in an inadequate oxygen supply can cause irregularities of the heartbeat that can end with cardiac arrest.

Recently, I was scheduled to perform a minor diagnostic surgical procedure for what I was sure was a benign condition on a patient who had a known irregular heart rhythm for which she was under the care of a cardiologist. She was taking a widely used medication for this problem. Although I wanted to perform the procedure using a local anesthetic, the patient, against my advice, was adamant. She felt that she would not be able to manage her fears and insisted on being put to sleep.

Before the patient was brought to the operating room, I discussed in detail the issues involved in her care with the anesthesiologist assigned to the outpatient surgical unit that day. I had never worked with this doctor before, but since I knew the procedure was straightforward, would take no more than thirty minutes, and the patient was essentially healthy, I was not overly concerned.

After the patient was asleep, as I prepped the surgical area and placed the sterile surgical drapes, I became aware that her heart rate had slowed from her resting rate of fifty-five to forty beats per minute. The video screen of the heart monitor was no longer a constant green, but was now blinking a cautionary yellow. With no alarm but some interest, I asked the anesthesiologist, "What's going on?"

She was initially defensive, thinking I was intruding on her turf. "Nothing serious," she insisted, somewhat peevishly. "Her basal rate is normally slow. She's on a beta blocker," she said, naming the drug the patient was using routinely as the cause for the marked slowing of her heart. I was not comfortable with that explanation.

"I tell you what, I'd like you to give her some atropine," I said, citing the drug that has been used for many years to increase the rate of a slowly beating heart.

She objected to what she belligerently characterized as my interference with her authority and prerogatives. Insisting that she did not like using atropine, she told me she would choose a different medication to correct the problem. I didn't care what she used. I just wanted to see the heart rate return to normal. The anesthesiologist administered a different drug. I decided to wait until the patient's heart rate had returned to normal before beginning the operation. The heart rate continued to slow, dropping quickly to thirty-three and then to thirty beats per minute. The heart monitor was now flashing red and an alarm went off alerting everyone to the possibility of a potentially catastrophic cardiac arrest. At this point, almost as concerned about my own rapidly increasing blood pressure, no longer willing to defer to this very junior physician, I insisted, "Give her some atropine now!"

It took another five minutes for the patient's heart rate to respond. Then slowly, over fifteen minutes, it returned to her normal resting rate. In the interim, after examining my options, I had decided not to proceed with the operation, since I could not be sure that she had not sustained some injury as a result of the lower heart rate and resultant reduced cardiac output. I was primarily concerned that were I to perform the planned surgery and she were to develop a similar episode of a dangerously low heart rate, it might not be as easily reversed and I would have to deal with a medical emergency.

I announced my decision, "I am not going to operate on her today," and explained why I had come to that conclusion. The anesthesiologist was angry. She knew there was nothing she could do about my canceling the procedure. I took this action knowing it would be equally unpopular with the patient. In fact, as it turned out, nothing bad had happened. I must say that even after a lot of explaining, the patient was sufficiently unhappy about my decision that I am sure if it were not for her cardiologist, who supported my action, she would have chosen to be cared for by another gynecologist.

If you have any illness on top of the one for which you're being operated on, anesthesia poses an even greater risk than usual. You should make every effort to avoid elective surgery if you have any other illnesses, including something as trivial as a cold. Even such a relatively minor problem as anemia can become a significant factor in a patient undergoing anesthesia.

It is clear that many deaths due to anesthesia are preventable. In many hospitals today, including major academic medical centers, certified registered nurse anesthetists deliver anesthesia to patients. Many board-certified anesthesiologists point to the less well trained nurse anesthetist as the root cause of deaths from anesthesia. While a nurse anesthetist may be competent to handle the majority, perhaps even 90 percent, of cases, it is the other 10 percent that can result in catastrophe.

There is no scarcity of anesthesiologists in America, and I would never allow anyone less than a highly qualified specialist physician to perform this vital and hazardous service. In my judgment, nurse anesthetists should work only under the direct and continuous supervision of a board-certified anesthesiologist. Since except in a true emergency, you cannot be put under anesthesia without signing a consent form, you should make your expectations clear with respect to the credentials that you require for the person who is going to administer anesthesia to you. Have this discussion before you're brought to the operating room.

This will be a great problem for senior citizens who participate in Medicare. The federal government, under plans initiated by President Clinton, as well as a substantial number of states are proposing plans that will permit nurse anesthetists to administer anesthesia to Medicare patients without physician supervision. Since these patients are more likely to have additional medical problems, I think it's courting disaster to permit this practice solely for the savings that would be generated by using nurses rather than physicians. Recent data documents that mortality rates increased by as much as 20 percent when nurse anesthetists worked without physician supervision. These new federal and state initiatives are being opposed by a variety of anesthesiologist organizations.

A significant issue with regard to this hospital-based service is the recognition that, contrary to the accepted law of physics that it is not possible to be in two different places at the same time, it is common practice in many hospitals for anesthesiologists to supervise the care for two and occasionally three or four patients who are undergoing surgery at the same time. In these cases, it is common practice for either a nurse anesthetist or anesthesiology resident-in-training to administer anesthesia while the attending anesthesiologist is caring for another patient in another operating room.

Spinal anesthesia, an alternative to general anesthesia where you are put to sleep, results in numbing only the surgical area. This technique involves the use of drugs administered into the spinal canal that block sensation of pain and inhibit muscle contraction below the level where the drugs are introduced into the spinal fluid. The drugs that are used for spinal anesthesia are not without risk, and can sometimes result in permanent paralysis, brain damage, and even death. More commonly, the ill effects of spinal anesthesia are headache, backache, and occasional nausea and vomiting.

If you choose this method, discuss it in advance with your surgeon and anesthesiologist. It is a procedure that requires skills that are only gained through experience. You want to be absolutely sure that your anesthesiologist has had this experience. As with all procedures involving instrumentation or medications, you should expect that the person in charge has had a few years of experience in their use. It is entirely appropriate for you to verify with the doctor that this is the case, and to put your requirements on the anesthesia consent form.

Regardless of the route or method of anesthesia or the drugs that are used, the risks do not end in the operating room. Close observation of the postoperative patient in the recovery room is critical and any negligence at this time can result in death. Most commonly, this period of care is supervised by nurses overseen by an anesthesiologist. You should be assured that the various electronic monitoring devices available will be used as you waken from anesthesia during the immediate postoperative period. These devices have built-in alarms that alert medical personnel in the recovery room if problems arise involving a patient's heart, blood pressure, or oxygen levels. These technologies are readily available. It is vital that you make sure that they are in place and are used in the recovery room of any hospital where you are going to be put under anesthesia for any reason. If they are not used routinely and you are facing an elective procedure, go to a hospital where they are standard procedure. You should address your questions about the recovery room routines to your surgeon as well as to the anesthesiologist.

While it is incumbent on you to specify your expectations with regard to the care and attention you will be given by the anesthesiologist, it is also appropriate for you to discuss these issues with your surgeon. You should be assured that these two physicians have reviewed your clinical situation in detail and each has discussed his or her plans of management with you. You should be fully informed about the anesthesia that will be used as well as the medications that you will receive for the control of postoperative pain. All these concerns and the details of who will provide you with this care should be fully described in writing on the consent form you sign.

Keep an Eye Out for Your Anesthesiologist

Carl Hart, the chief medical executive of a large managed care program, was on a trip to New Orleans, far from his home, when he thought he noticed a change in his eyesight. He described it as a blurring that involved a specific area in his field of vision. That Saturday night we were scheduled to have dinner together. We were at my home in the country when he told me what was happening. His symptoms were strongly suggestive of a retinal detachment that can lead to blindness, and therefore is a bona fide emergency. I insisted that we go to the emergency room of the local small community hospital. Although they were aware that their patient was a physician and held a position of substantial influence, the ER staff provided what I considered inadequate care. The ER physician decided not to call the ophthalmologist-on-call to the hospital to see this patient. In fact, the instrument to measure the pressure in the eye, the tonometer, was broken, so they could not rule out glaucoma, another possible, although unlikely, cause of the symptoms. They allowed Dr. Hart to leave the hospital without a diagnosis.

Less than thirty-six hours after we left the ER, Dr. Hart called me at my home to report that his symptoms had worsened. We had both returned to New York. I called a friend who is the chief of the eye service at a major teaching hospital whom I knew to be a world-class retinal surgeon. Within four hours, Dr. Hart had been diagnosed as having retinal detachments in both eyes. He was admitted to the hospital directly from the doctor's office. That evening he underwent an operation on his left eye. The procedure was uneventful.

The next day, Dr. Hart was brought to the operating room at four o'clock to have an operation on his right eye. After he had waited an interminable three hours on a gurney in the pre-anesthesia room, a doctor came to his side, picked up his chart, and began to read it. Dr. Hart asked, "Are you the anesthesiologist?"

There was a long pause before the man responded, "Ya. I'm Dr. ——." His name was unintelligible.

"I'm Carl Hart. I would like to talk with you for a minute."

The anesthesiologist stood with his chart in hand, saying nothing.

"You know I was operated on last night. I want you to know that everything went very well. I wasn't nauseated from the anesthetic and I really haven't had any significant pain since they took me back to my room last night."

The anesthesiologist simply nodded. Anyone lying on a gurney in a hospital gown is in a very dependent position. Dr. Hart's discomfiture prompted him to continue. "I would like you to use the same anesthetic." After a very long pause, the doctor simply nodded and walked away. This had hardly been a reassuring exchange. Dr. Hart was anxious when he was wheeled into the operating room.

The resident, an anesthesiologist-in-training, started Dr. Hart's intravenous line and hooked him up to the various monitors. It was July 2. Dr. Hart realized that if this resident was in his first year of training, he had had a total of two days of experience (see Chapter 2). He tried to calm himself by thinking about how flawlessly everything had gone the previous day.

Suddenly he realized that he was conscious and in pain. He was still in the operating room and his surgeon was still operating on his right eye. Dr. Hart felt as if his eye was being lifted partially out of the socket. He opened his left eye, vision blurred from the operation on the preceding day, and saw that the anesthesiology resident was alone. The attending, his instructor, was not in the room.

"Stop moving," the surgeon demanded.

As he tells it, Dr. Hart lost his cool and screamed. "Get the anesthesiologist back in this room. Put me to sleep." It took a few minutes. The next thing that he was aware of was being moved to the recovery room. He was retching and remained nauseated throughout the night.

Although all the specifics about the medications and anesthetic agents that had been used so successfully the day before were in the chart and readily available, it turned out the drugs used during the second operation were chosen by the resident who had not spoken to Dr. Hart before he was taken into the OR. These medications bore no relationship to what had been used the preceding day. When Dr. Hart learned that the second anesthesiologist had not managed him as he had been asked, he demanded to see the chief of the service. Because of his position as chief medical officer of a large insurance company, the chief of anesthesiology responded and came to his room before his discharge from the hospital. Dr. Hart was enraged and did not couch his anger. He believed that he had been ignored and told him, "If this is how you treat me, what can the average person expect when misfortune places him in your hands?"

The implicit contract between the patient and the anesthesiologist is a simple one. The doctor's obligation is to ensure that the patient gets through the procedure without pain and hopefully with some amnesia with respect to the experience. Unless you take steps ahead of time, you may meet your anesthesiologist for the first time just as you are about to enter the operating room. Except in an emergency, this is not appropriate care. It is essential that you discuss with your surgeon your very legitimate concerns with regard to this aspect of your care in detail and insist on meeting the anesthesiologist before you go to the OR.

At that meeting, before you sign the consent form, ask the following questions:

- Are you going to administer my anesthesia? If so, what is your name? (If not, who is? I have questions that I want to ask. When am I going to meet that person?)
- What is your position in the hospital? (The right answer is, "I'm an attending anesthesiologist.")
- What training have you had? (The right answer is, "I have completed a residency in anesthesiology.")
- Are you a board-certified anesthesiologist? (There is no reason for you not to be provided the services of a board-certified anesthesiologist. The right answer is, yes. If the doctor has recently completed residency training, he or she will not yet be board-certified. If the answer is no, and their residency was finished more than three years ago, you should be concerned. Did the doctor take the board exam and fail? Or decide not to take it at all? You may not

get an honest answer to the questions that naturally flow from this information.)

- Are you intending to be in the operating room from the beginning to the end of my surgery? (Yes is the right answer. Except for being relieved when necessary by another equally well-trained anesthesiologist, to ensure continuity of care you want an anesthesiologist to take you all the way through the surgical procedure.)
- Will you supervise my care in the recovery room? (In many hospitals, the transition from the OR to the recovery room results in the anesthesiologist passing the baton to a colleague. In the hospital, every time there is a change of shifts in the hospital with a change in personnel, there is an increased probability of a mistake being introduced in your care. The move from the OR to the recovery room is a particularly risky transition. You should make it clear to your surgeon that you expect him or her to be involved in this process.)

In such circumstances, when you are operated on and have received anesthesia, you are going to be billed and you and/or your insurance carrier will have to pay for the services of an attending anesthesiologist. It is therefore only reasonable that you receive the care and services for which you are paying. It is your obligation and responsibility to ensure that this happens. The consent form is the formal document of your assignment of this responsibility. When you are asked to sign the anesthesia consent form, it is both appropriate and necessary for you to document in writing your expectations with regard to the supervision of the anesthesia that you will be given. There is a section on every consent form that you are asked to sign that is customarily labeled "Restrictions," where you are free to write the specifications that you want to have followed. This can include the name of the anesthesiologist as well as any other requirements. Insist that your anesthesia be delivered by a board-certified anesthesiologist, and that he or she be present for the entire operation unless relieved by another doctor *with equivalent credentials.*

Radiologists

The radiologist, another hospital-based physician, is often a pivotal figure in your care even though you almost never get to choose him or her. While it has become common for patients, when faced with significant medical problems, to ask for a second opinion, I cannot recall a single instance of a patient asking me to secure an independent review of an X-ray, CAT scan, or MRI, the domain of the radiologist, even though many medical and surgical interventions are undertaken based on the interpretation of such studies.

David Solomon was a healthy fifty-five-year-old CEO of a Fortune 500 company when he first noticed an intermittent and occasionally severe pain radiating down his right leg. After self-medicating with aspirin for several weeks, he called his internist who had been caring for his minor ailments for more than ten years. He was referred to a prominent orthopedist who was director of the service at a prestigious hospital. The doctor's secretary gave him an appointment for the following week.

By the time he was seen, the pain was more intense and the episodes more frequent. After what he described as a perfunctory interview and a brief focused examination, he was dispatched with a prescription for a nonsteroidal anti-inflammatory medicine from the Advil family, a diagnosis of "sciatica," and told to return in two months.

Things did not improve, but Solomon was a very busy man and he attempted first to dismiss and then deny his symptoms. He rationalized that he had seen a reputable, highly respected physician, been given medicine, and told to come back in two months. Still, four weeks before he was to return, I noticed that he was walking with a very unusual gait.

One week later, he was clearly disabled. I broached the subject with him. He had developed a foot drop and had lost proprioception—the ability to sense where a part of your body is. He only knew where his right foot was when he looked at it. The pain hadn't gone away. It was clear that he had substantial damage to the nerves in his leg. I suggested that he needed immediate attention and told him he was seeing the wrong specialist. I thought he would be better served by a neurologist. Like most patients, he was concerned that were he to follow my suggestion it would offend both his internist and the orthopedist. I was able to persuade him to call the orthopedist for an immediate appointment and to have a CAT scan.

I was not surprised when Solomon told me that he thought the orthopedist was perturbed at the suggestion that the scan be done but had agreed to order it. He saw no reason for advancing the date of the follow-up visit. The scan was done the following week. The week after that, the patient called the orthopedist to hear the report. His secretary called back later that day and reported that the scan was normal.

By the following week, Solomon was unable to walk to his office and now had his chauffeur pick him up at the beginning and the end of each day. At the time of his scheduled follow-up examination, the orthopedist decided that he needed a two-week course of steroids. By chance, I saw Solomon that evening. By now he was clearly upset by his obvious disability and was able to begin to express some irritation with the doctor, who he felt was not sufficiently attentive. I volunteered to help.

The following morning I went to the radiology department of the hospital where the scan had been done. After getting his films from the X-ray file room, I went to the neuroradiology reading room. The radiology resident, a doctor-in-training who had originally read the scan, was there. I reviewed the films with him. There had been no mistake. The scan was entirely normal. There was, however, a problem. The scan had not included the lower part of the spine, which was the probable site of the source of the problems.

The requisition for the scan that his orthopedist's secretary had given to a secretary at the radiology department over the phone was incomplete. Neither the radiology technician who had done the study nor the radiologist interpreting the scan had a thorough understanding of the patient's clinical history. Functionally, they had no idea why the procedure was being done. As a result of this miscommunication and the failure to transmit the patient's complete and relevant history, the technician took the wrong series of X-rays.

The interpretation of an X-ray is a subjective matter. An accurate reading is only possible when the radiologist knows the patient's history. Had the radiologist known the patient's history, he would have recognized that the wrong X-ray study had been done.

I explained the problem to the resident. He called the attending neuroradiologist on duty. It was agreed that the patient should be brought back and the appropriate scan be done as soon as possible. They were all properly embarrassed and concerned.

I called David Soloman at his office and told him exactly

what had happened. I suggested that he come back as soon as possible to have the scan done. He arrived at the CAT scan suite fifteen minutes later.

One hour later, the proper radiological study had been completed and the diagnosis made. Soloman had a slipped disc that was impinging on his spinal cord. This was the source of his symptoms.

A week later, Soloman was admitted to another hospital and was operated on by a neurosurgeon who removed the offending disc. After a two-day postoperative stay and an additional ten days of convalescence, he returned to a schedule of limited physical activity. One month later, he was able to resume all normal activities, including tennis. Due to the damage the nerves had sustained as a result of the prolonged compression by the disc, the muscles of the leg had become atrophied. It took an additional ten months for him to regain normal strength in his right leg.

Soloman's anger at having received what he characterized as "third-rate care" has not diminished to this day. He had lived with the conviction that by virtue of his wealth, position, and power, he would be assured of first-class medical care. This episode permanently undermined this assumption.

Ask your physician if he or she has reviewed your X-rays and discussed them with the radiologist who is responsible for the official interpretation. Your medical care is inadequate if this hasn't been done.

Every test your physician orders should be done for a good reason. It is your physician who should explain the results of these studies and what is to follow. It is important that you take the initiative to impress on him or her the need for unceasing vigilance in the information-gathering process as you go from diagnosis to treatment. If at any point, you or your physician are not entirely comfortable with what you are being told by any consultant such as a radiologist, it is reasonable, indeed necessary, for you to request a second expert opinion. You and your physician must join forces if there's any issue with regard to payment by the managed care organization for such second opinions.

Pathologists

It is difficult if not impossible not to be anxious while waiting for the results of a biopsy regardless of the organ involved. Your ultimate diagnosis is often made based on the pathologist's interpretation of the microscopic appearance of the cells obtained from biopsies and smears. And it is based on this opinion that treatment plans are made and procedures performed.

A search of the medical literature confirms the conclusion that the diagnostic discrepancy rate for pathology specimens is sufficiently high that a second opinion is often not only justified but, if logistically possible, strongly indicated. In a startling number of cases, this second review led the first pathologist to revise his or her original opinion, downgrading, for example, an invasive cancer to a much less dire condition.

Time and again, I have seen patients who have undergone extensive surgery as a result of erroneous pathologic diagnoses. Rarely have I had a patient who has asked for a second opinion of a positive Pap smear or breast biopsy. If there is a discrepancy between the independent interpretations of any pathology specimen, there is no question that the cost of such additional reviews should be paid by most insurance carriers, though you may have to do battle to have such service covered. (A discussion of the general principles of tackling such a task are fully discussed in Chapter 1.)

* * *

My patient was only thirteen years old when a mass was discovered in her right ovary. She arrived in my office for a second opinion when surgery was recommended and the specter of cancer was raised after a thorough preoperative workup. I told her anxious parents that there was no doubt about the need for surgery. The diagnosis of ovarian cancer could only be made at the time of surgery. For a variety of reasons, they decided that I should operate on their daughter. Preoperatively, I explained to them that I would not be able to tell them exactly what was going to be done in the operating room. Depending upon what I found, it was possible that I would be forced to do a hysterectomy and remove both ovaries.

During the operation, there was no question that the patient had a very large tumor that had essentially destroyed her right ovary. I removed it. Although it appeared normal, as a precaution I took a biopsy of her left ovary. The specimens were sent out for what is known as a "frozen section." The pathologist quickly prepares the tissue by literally freezing and processing the specimen and gives the surgeon a preliminary diagnosis. In ten minutes I was given an ominous diagnosis that, if valid, required that I remove the remaining ovary and uterus.

I was uncomfortable with what I had been told and felt that the pathologist assigned to do the frozen sections in the OR that day was quite junior. In view of the discrepancy between my clinical opinion and the pathologist's frozen section diagnosis, I decided to wait for the interpretation of what are called the "permanent sections" of the tissue. I closed the patient's abdomen and told her family that it was possible that their daughter would have to undergo additional, definitive surgery.

Over the course of the next week, dozens of slides were

made from the patient's surgical specimens and reviewed by several senior pathologists. After much debate, they decided to ask the opinion of other highly qualified pathologists. The patient's slides were sent to a famous surgical pathologist in Boston and another at the Armed Forces Institute of Pathology in Washington. Finally, the decision was made that the patient's tumor was not malignant, her left ovary was healthy, and she required no further surgery.

While this is not a typical case in terms of the complexity of the diagnosis, it is a very good example of the pivotal issues that rest on the shoulders of the pathologist. I could cite literally hundreds of cases in my experience where the wrong thing was done based solely on the microscopic interpretation of a single slide. These errors include instances where the wrong procedure was performed, an unnecessary operation was done, as well as where nothing was done and subsequently a reevaluation of a slide resulted in a change in the diagnosis from a benign lesion to cancer.

It is important that you understand the role of the pathologist. As the explosive growth of knowledge has driven the development of the many medical subspecialties, a similar general class of specialization has developed in pathology. There are pathologists who specialize in dermatology, obstetrics and gynecology, pediatrics, and surgery. You should make every effort to ensure that you obtain the opinion of one who is highly qualified, and have an independent second opinion when a critical clinical decision rests on any potentially problematic diagnosis.

Outpatient Care

It is increasingly likely that when you are ill you will go to the hospital for testing with high-tech X-rays and/or be treated as an outpatient. More and more surgical procedures are being done on an outpatient basis. This is in large part due to the new technologies that permit what is commonly known as minimally invasive surgery. Even procedures that historically have required inpatient hospitalization are now being performed on an outpatient basis. While there has been a great deal of criticism of outpatient surgery and short hospital stays, it has been shown that, in the proper setting, this is not only appropriate but better care.

Outpatient Tests—Who Does What? Who Decides What It All Means?

I recently underwent a series of tests including an MRI and an electromyelogram (EMG), with nerve conduction studies of my arm and hand. Initially, when I arrived at the EMG laboratory, a technician was assigned to perform the test. After asking a few questions, the technician left the room and a more senior neurology fellow came in, introduced himself, and told me he would perform the test. I'd been given a medical upgrade! I asked, "Why the change?" He was clearly uncomfortable but admitted it was because I was a physician on the staff of the hospital. I was amused because I had thought the technician probably had more experience and was in all likelihood more proficient in performing the test. However, I did not object.

After two hours of testing, some of which was quite uncomfortable, I asked the fellow to review the results with me. He was most deferential and spent more than thirty minutes going over them and giving me his interpretation. Since I am not a neurologist, I was just a bit more at home with him than I am when talking to an automobile mechanic about the fuel injection system in my car.

It was two weeks later that my neurologist, who had ordered the test, faxed the official interpretation to me and called me in order to review the results. He was, at first, irritated and quite critical of the written report that he had received, since it was couched with many conditional clauses and ended with "a repeat study could be done in three to six months if clinically indicated." Asserting his authority, he told me, "I know damn well what's wrong. I wrote a very detailed requisition to them. Their test just didn't demonstrate it."

It was only then that I interrupted him. "Wait a second, Bob. The written report is really quite different from what the neurology fellow told me when we went over the results together."

Indeed, there was a significant discrepancy between the two interpretations. With this information, my neurologist was even more exercised. Over the next three days, he tried to get some clarification from the EMG lab. It was only after many telephone calls that he was able to confront the director of the lab about the differences between what I had been told and what had been written. After all his efforts, we were both left in the position of having a test with an ambiguous result.

The point of this story is that when you are undergoing any test, make sure you know who will interpret the results and how and to whom they will be reported and by whom they will be reviewed. This demands that you maintain a level of attention and a proactive stance. My experience as well as David Solomon's demonstrate the need to review the results of any test with your physician.

Although it is intellectually and emotionally difficult to accept, errors in medicine are not uncommon. This episode highlights the point that as things become more and more complex, the likelihood of error increases. Medical error is, most commonly, not the result of malice or greed. While it is reasonable to make every effort to reduce the probability of error, it will never be possible to reduce it to zero. You must remain alert. Don't passively accept any recommendation without a full explanation of all its potential implications.

Whenever errors have been made and are uncovered, there is usually no issue with regard to the payment for repeating the studies. However, this is another issue where you are totally dependent on your physician. It is his or her vigilance and attention to detail that will minimize the likelihood of your being exposed to untoward results—and the attendant costs—that come from decisions based on flawed data.

A reflection of the risks involved in being a patient is revealed by the establishment of the National Patient Safety Foundation by the American Medical Association in partnership with several other interested organizations. This group is providing the funding for projects that will evaluate methods to improve patient safety. Offering grants of up to $100,000, this organization has highlighted the increasing incidence of errors that have resulted in significant complications for patients.

If you are to undergo any test—ranging from having a needle put in your vein or a catheter placed in your bladder to a procedure with some risk, such as a heart stress test—you must understand that your questions are not unreasonable. It is astonishing that people who will question extensively every other person with whom they do business of even the most trivial sort often will abdicate any responsibility about medical matters of such importance. I believe in many cases this is a function of patients' deference to the authoritative physician and fear of offending a person on whom they know they are so dependent.

Ask the following questions before undergoing any test:

- Why is this test being done?
- What can it possibly show or prove that you don't know now?
- Who is going to perform the test?
- What are the risks of the test?
- Who will manage a complication if it occurs?
- When will I be told the results of the test?
- Who will give, tell, and/or show me the results?
- Will you, my physician, review the results with me? When?

If you don't get satisfactory answers, say so and ask for a more detailed discussion of why your physician believes that you should undergo this test and how the results will be of use in the management of your problem. Until and unless this all makes sense to you, you must continue to search for reasonable answers to your questions.

CHAPTER 4

Procedures: Why, When, and Where

Have you ever noticed how much quieter people are inside an airplane that is taking off or landing than when you have reached the cruising altitude? Think about it. Everyone knows takeoffs and landings are when there is the greatest risk of a mishap. It is this unstated recognition of risk that inhibits conversation. Although much of the practice of medicine is like flying at forty thousand feet, from personal experience, I assure you that performing a procedure is like constantly taking off and landing.

When you give someone a hammer, it is natural for him or her to look for a nail. For physicians who have taken the time and made the effort to develop the skills to perform a highly technical, complex procedure, it is to be expected that they look forward to the opportunity to practice their highly demanding craft. From personal experience, I can tell you this is true, and when a relatively large fee for performing the procedure is added to the equation, it would be beyond belief to expect that someone would not look hard to find patients who need the procedure. As a result of the increasing number of physicians and the effects of the fee schedules of managed care organizations, many physicians have seen a reduction in their income. With this in mind, you should be very clear as to why your physician is recommending you undergo any procedure. Just about every problem has one or more alternative, competitive treatment approaches. It is very important that your physician thoroughly review all the options with you. Every procedure, no matter how simple it appears, has associated risks, and none is performed with uniform expertise by all practitioners. Without exception, if the opportunity is available, I recommend you get a second opinion.

One need not necessarily adhere to the belief that "in life, timing is everything," but there is ample evidence that this concept has great merit with regard to the timing of medical procedures. As I mentioned in the hospital chapter, procedures are classified as emergent, urgent, and elective. If you're hemorrhaging and treatment must begin within minutes or you'll suffer irreversible damage or death, it's an emergency and there is, in effect, no time to carefully research and evaluate your options. If you have an urgent problem, it requires attention but can wait a matter of hours or even a few days. An elective procedure is one that can be handled safely at your or your physician's convenience. The question of when to schedule urgent or elective procedures is a significant issue.

Fortunately, the majority of medical procedures can be scheduled electively. This works to your advantage, since a procedure done as an emergency has a greater likelihood of complication than one done electively.

Even with the same doctor, in the same hospital, a procedure done in the middle of the night as an emergency never runs as smoothly as when everyone knows in advance what time the patient will arrive in the operating room. The medical literature is filled with articles to support the assertion that the outcome of any procedure is in part a function of when it is done—the day of the week, the time of day, the proximity to major holidays, and, in teaching hospitals, the month of the year! All surgical procedures have risks. Even with no other medical problems, the patient risks infection, hemorrhage, inadvertent injury to internal organs, delayed wound healing, and even death. It is because of these risks that I echo my mentors when I say "There is no such thing as minor surgery, only minor surgeons."

If It's Not an Emergency Don't Have It Done Outside of Normal Working Hours

Ms. Deborah Lynette's problem was considered somewhat urgent. Because there was no open time on the operating room schedule for the following morning, and her surgeon had planned a round of golf the next afternoon, for his convenience he persuaded the chief OR nurse to add her to the operating room schedule. Ms. Lynette would be done at the end of the day after all the scheduled cases had been completed. By the time her surgeon was notified that a room with the necessary staff had become available, it was already early evening. By the time she was brought into the operating room, it was almost nine P.M.

Everything was going exactly as the surgeon had planned. He was close to finishing the technically difficult part of the procedure when the OR nursing supervisor came into the room. Following OR etiquette, she asked the surgeon, "May I speak with you, Dr. Warren?"

Turning away from the table, he said, "Yes, of course."

"It appears there is a problem here."

Since as far as Dr. Warren was concerned, everything was going along as he expected, he was puzzled. "Everything's fine here. What's up?"

"I'm afraid that the tray of instruments you are using isn't sterile."

"What?" He knew exactly what she had said. He knew exactly what it meant. He couldn't believe what he had just been told.

"There was a cart full of used instrument trays in the corridor that were to be taken down for sterilization. When the instrument tray was requisitioned for this room the transporter made a mistake and took a tray from that cart and gave it to the circulating nurse. The circulator didn't notice that the tray wasn't sealed and therefore not sterile. There was a change in the scrub nurse assigned to this room at that time and the new scrub nurse thought the instrument tray you were using had been opened by the nurse she had relieved. We just discovered what happened when the trays were counted."

Dr. Warren was livid. He had been operating on this patient for the past two hours using nonsterile instruments. He thought "Hepatitis, AIDS, God only knows what!" There was absolutely nothing that he could do about what had happened, about the unnecessary risks to which his patient had been exposed. The probability of these errors is far higher when conditions aren't routine.

Stay Out of the OR on Friday Afternoon— a Difference of Life and Death

The outcome for Helen Robinson demonstrates the importance of timing for elective surgery. Mrs. Robinson was a fifty-year-old, slightly overweight woman who required a vaginal hysterectomy with repair of her bladder and rectum as a result of a condition known as pelvic relaxation. The operation was necessary because the patient had frequent episodes of urinary incontinence and occasionally lost stool when she passed gas. Its timing, however, was elective. The operation was scheduled to be done on a Friday afternoon by a gynecologist with an academic appointment in a teaching hospital.

This was a routine surgical procedure for Dr. Stone, a surgeon who had a great deal of experience performing this operation on patients who were considered to be at normal risk. The morning of the day following surgery, the patient had many complaints, which she told the resident on morning rounds, summing up with "I really feel crummy." Her husband arrived when visiting hours began at noon. He was concerned about his wife's appearance. Assuming her doctor had seen her earlier in the day, and hoping to get some reassurance that everything was as expected, he asked her, "What did Dr. Stone have to say?" It was only then that he learned "He's away for the weekend. His associate came in this morning and told me everything is fine."

Early on Sunday morning, the patient developed shaking chills and a fever. There was no question about it; she had an infection. After the resident consulted with the physician covering for Dr. Stone, Mrs. Robinson was started on several antibiotics. She was not feeling any better Sunday afternoon. In the late afternoon, her husband called the doctor who was taking Dr. Stone's calls. When he got that physician on the phone, he reported, "My wife really looks terrible." At this point he learned that he was talking to a physician who had never seen his wife. The doctor who had been covering for Dr. Stone on Saturday was unavailable and had "signed out" to this doctor. Mr. Robinson was told, "I'm sure she's doing as expected. You don't have a lot of experience in seeing patients who have just had major surgery. I'm sure if there was anything to be concerned about I would hear about it from the resident. In any event, Dr. Stone will be back in the morning."

At six o'clock on Monday morning, the resident was called by the nurse who reported there was a marked change in Mrs. Robinson's vital signs. Her temperature had risen to 104, her blood pressure had fallen, and her heart rate had increased. These were unmistakable signs that she had a widely disseminated infection. This can be a life-threatening complication of surgery. The resident called Dr. Stone at his home. When he arrived in her room at 7:00 A.M., Dr. Stone recognized immediately that something was very seriously wrong. He made arrangements for Mrs. Robinson to be moved to the surgical intensive care unit. She died later that day.

When a patient who has recently undergone surgery dies unexpectedly, the case becomes the province of the medical examiner and a detailed investigation is carried out. An autopsy revealed that Mrs. Robinson had developed an overwhelming infection with an organism that was not sensitive to the antibiotics that were being used. This infection had progressed to septic shock that led to her death. The autopsy proved that the root cause of her death was due to an error that took place during the operation. It revealed that she had sustained two completely separate intra-operative injuries. Her right ureter, the tube that carries urine from the right kidney to the bladder, had been cut and tied. In addition, she had a small hole in her large intestine that had permitted spillage of fecal material into her abdominal cavity and caused a fulminating infectious peritonitis. Both of these inadvertent injuries have been made by many good surgeons over the course of a working life-time. In fact, many surgeons would say that if a surgeon hasn't experienced one of the known complications of the operation he or she is performing, it is because he or she hasn't done enough of them.

The fault here lies not in making the surgical error but in not recognizing it and, more significantly, compounding the error by inattention to the many, many symptoms Mrs. Robinson exhibited over the forty-eight hours following the surgery. By Friday night, just six hours after the operation had been completed, this patient's hospital record contained ample evidence to justify taking her back to the operating room and opening her abdomen. In the absence of that, she certainly deserved a workup for her fever and evaluation of the pain she was experiencing, which was recorded in detail in the nurse's notes.

By Saturday at noon, the results of the blood tests that had been ordered clearly supported the conclusion that she had a significant infection. She had blood and pus in her urine and her clinical course was deviating markedly from what could reasonably be expected for a woman who had undergone a vaginal hysterectomy and surgical repair of her bladder and rectum. Still nothing was done. Saturday evening, she was being seen by a different resident, the fourth responsible for her care since she left the OR, who was reporting to the attending who was covering Dr. Stone's practice. The resident had called the covering attending after she had seen Mrs. Robinson when her temperature was recorded as 104.8 orally. This was eight hours after she had been started on broad-spectrum antibiotics.

She was not seen again by a physician for more than twelve hours. During that time her vital signs had progressively deteriorated, providing even more glaring evidence of the disaster that was to follow. By early Monday morning,

186 / O<small>UTSMARTING</small> M<small>ANAGED</small> C<small>ARE</small>

her blood pressure had fallen and she was in shock. When she was transferred to the ICU, the trajectory of her course was such that her death was probably inevitable, although even then it might have been possible to save her.

The most striking feature of Mrs. Robinson's unfortunate course was that from the time she left the operating room, she was never seen by the same physician more than once, and until Monday morning when Dr. Stone returned to the hospital, she was not seen by any physician who had taken part in the operation.

If something goes wrong in a postoperative patient, it is more than likely because the surgeon did something wrong, and very often it will take additional surgery to fix it. The person most likely to recognize a surgical complication is the doctor who performed the surgery. The problem here, without doubt, was the absence of any continuity of care for Mrs. Robinson. It is your right and the physician's obligation to ensure that this is provided.

I must admit that my own obsessive-compulsive personality has prohibited me from delegating the postoperative care of my patients to another physician. I believe I'm better informed about what I've done and have the most well-grounded view of what my patients should "look" like on post-op day one, two, and so on. Although this practice of following my patients in the postoperative period circumscribed my social life, my patients were impressed by my dedication. I am also convinced it was one of the most significant elements of my practice in terms of patients referring other patients to me for surgery. I firmly believe that my patients did better because of it.

Clearly, there have to be patients whose operations are scheduled for Friday afternoon. However, if you are to have elective surgery and your operation is set for a Friday afternoon, try to have it changed. If that's not possible, it is absolutely essential for you to know, in advance, exactly who will supervise your care during the crucial forty-eight to seventy-two hours following surgery. Not only do you want to know the names and ways to contact the physicians who will be responsible for your care, it's a good idea for you to meet these doctors in advance of your surgery.

Who Will Be There When You Need Help?

Another issue to consider in timing a procedure involves the need for additional consultants. If you are going to have a screening colonoscopy by a gastroenterologist to rule out cancer of the colon, a procedure that is being done with increasing frequency every year, you should be aware that one of the known complications of the procedure is perforation of the colon. Should perforation of the colon occur, major surgery is required to repair it. So you'll want to be sure that if such a complication does happen that the appropriate surgeon will be available. Here is a situation where an elective procedure, the colonoscopy, has the potential for causing problems that could require urgent and at times emergent attention. Before undergoing any procedure, discuss with your physician the potential problems that can arise and determine the appropriate time and place for undergoing the procedure. Don't schedule a procedure if the back-up staff won't be available.

The availability of hospital staff during the postoperative period is another consideration when planning the time of day and day of the week for elective procedures. This is demonstrated by the case of Mrs. Priscilla Reynolds.

Mrs. Reynolds was operated on in the afternoon. Her elective surgery was uneventful, and although she had underlying heart and lung disease, the internist who had supervised her preoperative medical care and the surgeon were satisfied after they jointly evaluated her condition upon her transfer to the recovery room. Together they went to her room to give a report to her waiting family.

One half hour after her arrival in the recovery room, during a change in the nursing shift, she had a respiratory arrest. Because she wasn't attached to an oxygen monitor, it went unnoticed until it resulted in a change in her heart-beat, which was detected by the cardiac monitor. After the alarm sounded, she was successfully resuscitated.

Regrettably, as a result of a prolonged period without adequate oxygen, Mrs. Reynolds had suffered substantial brain damage. She remained alive without regaining con-sciousness for many years before she died. As a result of her death, the hospital purchased additional oxygen sensors and used them on every patient recovering from anesthesia. This technology provides an early warning of a drop in the postoperative patient's oxygen level long before any significant problem occurs.

The fundamental point of these stories is that many people are involved in the care of any patient who has un-dergone a procedure. While it comes as a surprise to most people, the operating room and the recovery room are not isolated from changes in working personnel during coffee breaks, meal times, and the changing of shifts. In fact, when an operation goes beyond the end of a shift, there will be a change in many of the personnel in the operating room, in-cluding, at the very least, the scrub nurse who works at the surgeon's side, and the circulating nurse, whose job in-volves the ongoing supplying of the operating room with needed instruments and supplies. There may also be a change in the anesthesiologist and the surgical assistants.

Such changes in personnel inevitably affect the continuity and pace of the procedure. These same changes occur in the recovery room and result in the passage of the baton from one nurse who is going off duty to the new nurse who will take over the care of the patient in the immediate postoperative recovery period. As with any other similar situation, there are inevitable changes of staff at the end of the workday throughout the hospital. These logistics should be an integral part of your decision-making process when deciding the timing of any elective procedure.

Everything else being equal, it is better to be the first operative case of the day and to be operated on earlier rather than later in the week. Once scheduled, it's not usually possible to have the time of your operation changed. You can, however, if you are willing to wait, tell your surgeon that you want, for example, to be the first case on a Monday or Tuesday. What is also very important is that you make sure that your surgeon has not planned a vacation just before or immediately following your scheduled operation.

Unless You Don't Have a Choice, Stay Out of the Hospital in July

In addition to consideration of the time of day and day of the week when scheduling elective procedures, it is also important to understand that July 1 is "moving up day" in every academic medical center and teaching hospital in this country. On this day, all of the doctors-in-training change their positions in the hierarchy of medicine and assume increased clinical responsibility. This transition is marked by confusion and is fertile ground for problems and errors, all of which can affect your care.

Dr. Lloyd Warren was the intern on the medical ward at six o'clock on Friday of the Fourth of July weekend. It was his first night on duty as a physician after graduation from medical school. Everyone free to leave the hospital had left. Dr. Warren had responsibility for forty patients. His immediate superior, a first-year resident, Martin Carmody, was in charge of twice that number. John Booker, the chief resident, was in charge of twice that number plus those patients in the medical ICU. That night, every patient on the medical service was dependent on someone who was new to his job. While Drs. Carmody and Booker had some experience, that is very, very different from having been in a job and feeling as comfortable as possible about what you will be called upon to do.

Mr. Greenbaum, a barrel-chested man of sixty-five, arrived on the floor reporting that he hadn't been feeling well since lunch. He had tried all afternoon to get in touch with his physician, but since it was the Fourth of July weekend, his calls went unanswered. When the answering service informed him that the office was closed for the weekend, he decided to go directly to the emergency room.

Dr. Warren took his history and did a physical examination. Although he found several things wrong with Mr. Greenbaum, there was nothing he thought was acute. One of the problems he heard was the murmur of aortic stenosis. The aortic valve is the gate between the pumping chamber of the heart and the major artery that carries blood to the rest of the body. If that gate doesn't open fully, the flow of blood through the aortic valve will make a murmuring sound. The heart has to work harder to push the blood through the smaller opening so there is a higher pressure inside the pumping chamber. Over time, this higher pressure is transmitted back into the lungs. When this happens, fluid can leak out of the blood vessels and into the lungs;

this is called pulmonary edema. It's like drowning, but instead of water coming from outside in, the fluid moves from inside the blood vessels and fills the lungs. The patient with pulmonary edema reacts just like a drowning man. He becomes frantic, terrified, fighting, gasping for a breath of air.

When he listened to Mr. Greenbaum's lungs, Dr. Warren thought he heard the sound of a little fluid at the base of the left lung. It was a significant sign, but he decided not seriously threatening. He questioned his patient closely. "Well, Doc, I know there is something wrong with my heart. I've had that problem for four, no, five years. But my doctor told me it's not serious. He gave me two medicines. I ran out of them a few months ago and I haven't had a chance to get back to him. Matter of fact, I really don't feel any different when I'm taking them and they make me pee like a faucet. I can't even see a movie from beginning to end without having to go to the men's room. When I'm taking them, I can't get a good night's sleep. I'm up at least once and sometimes twice during the night."

Dr. Warren wrote the admitting note and paged his resident, Dr. Carmody, to discuss Mr. Greenbaum's management and the orders. From Carmody's tone, it was clear that he had his hands full, and before he could finish, the resident interrupted him, "Look, I have a bunch of sick people on my hands. This guy doesn't sound like he even belongs in the hospital. Get bloods, chest X-ray, EKG, and put him to bed. Start an IV with dextrose and water at a rate just to keep the vein open. If everything looks okay forget about him." Carmody was under the stress of his newly assumed responsibilities and didn't appreciate that Warren was not up to the task of focusing his attention on the potential problems of a patient with Mr. Greenbaum's history or current complaints.

"I've done all that," Warren assured him.

Dr. Warren then made several suggestions but Dr. Carmody put him off. "I'll come down to review it with you when I have a spare minute."

At 1:30 A.M., as could have been predicted, and what the right medication would probably have prevented, Mr. Greenbaum went into acute respiratory distress. His heart was racing and his lungs had filled with fluid halfway up on both sides. There was no question he was developing florid pulmonary edema, a life-threatening condition. Dr. Warren told the nurses to get the oxygen apparatus. He administered morphine, digitalis, and a diuretic. But he knew he needed help and he paged the resident. Dr. Carmody, who had just finished his first year of training, was fully occupied with a patient who had just suffered cardiac arrest. He was new to the job of supervising the management of a patient whose heart had stopped beating. He told Dr. Warren that if he really needed help he should call Dr. Booker, the chief resident.

"Really need help? Are you crazy? What do you think I put out a stat page for?" Dr. Warren put in a call for Booker.

The operator said, "He's on another call. Do you want to wait?"

"No. Interrupt him and tell him this is an emergency." Dr. Booker got on the phone.

"John, I'm in deep trouble. I have a sixty-five-year-old guy who has just gone into pulmonary edema. I'm alone with just a student and Carmody is tied up."

The chief resident was sympathetic but he was also being pressed. "I have a guy up here in shock pouring blood out of every orifice. Tell me what you are doing for your patient."

After meticulously detailing every step he planned to take, Dr. Warren asked, "Doesn't this guy belong in the ICU?"

"Probably does. But I don't have a bed free and there's

no one I can ship out right now." Booker did not want to be forced to make a decision about moving someone out of the intensive care unit. The downside possibilities of such a decision were significant. "It sounds to me that you have everything under control. Give me a call in half an hour and let's see where we all stand then."

"John, you have got to be kidding."

"No, Lloyd, I am not. You're the only horse, so I'm betting on you. Now get to it. It will be a terrific learning experience for you. Talk to you later." With that, the line went dead.

As he went back to his patient, Dr. Warren wondered what kind of a learning experience it would be for Mr. Greenbaum. Through the night, he did what he thought was right and what was necessary. He realized that he was "flying by the seat of his pants." It was 6:30 A.M. when Mr. Greenbaum finally regained full consciousness and opened his eyes. The sun had cleared the horizon. There was a bright blue sky.

"It going to be a nice day, Doc. You saved my life. I know I'm here today because of you. Thanks."

Lloyd Warren smiled. He knew what his patient had said was true. He knew that he would never forget this experience, this first night on call. Without a doubt, this was the first person whose life he had truly saved.

Every physician will recall and relish the chance to share the details of their Mr. Greenbaums with you. When you ask when that event occurred, it was invariably in July or at the latest August in the first year of their training. And then they may privately recall the patients for whom they also cared at an early stage of their training for whom the outcome was not so positive.

The problems that occur to patients in teaching hospitals in July and August each year are much more likely to be resolved slowly or with difficulty or not satisfactorily than those that are dealt with later in the training year. Don't schedule any elective admission to a teaching hospital in July or August if you can avoid it.

Pick a Physically and Mentally Fit Doctor

For the surgeon, an operation is a physical as well as a cerebral undertaking. Many of my own patients, as they are being prepared by the anesthesiologist on the operating table, look up at me and ask, "Did you have a good night's sleep, Doctor?" or "You weren't out at a party drinking last night were you, Doctor?" or "You're not tired, are you, Doctor?" These are not unreasonable questions, and in many instances are quite appropriate. You might even ask, "How are things between you and your significant other?"

There is no doubt that fatigue can affect surgical performance. It is appropriate for the patient who is to be the third case on the doctor's schedule, after the surgeon has already spent four or five or six hours in surgery that day, to be concerned that the surgeon may no longer be at the top of his or her form. You should ask what case you are on the surgeon's schedule and what time the operation will be done. Don't be that third patient!

I can tell you from personal experience that it takes a lot of insight for a surgeon to acknowledge his or her own physical limitations, and courage not to be so caught up in the system to be daunted by the institutional and personal consequences of canceling an operation. I can recall three instances where I had four cases scheduled in one day and as a result of unanticipated complications in the earlier cases felt it was the better part of wisdom not to undertake the last case on my schedule. I canceled those procedures after speaking with the patients and candidly telling them of my concerns. They were all very understanding and accepted my decision with grace. Of course, it would be the unusual person who would want to be operated on by a tired surgeon.

There is one instance in my own career that made the point of just how fragile one's level of performance can be. Between my first and second cases, I received a telephone call informing me that my ninety-nine-year-old father had died. I thought about canceling the scheduled operation but the patient was already in the operating room and the anesthesia had been started. Since it was an operation that I had done literally hundreds of times without incident, I decided to go ahead as planned. Midway through the procedure, I got into difficulty and the patient suffered an inadvertent injury. It was recognized and repaired, but the patient required a lengthy procedure and a prolonged hospitalization. This happened almost ten years ago. To this day, when I think about my father, that patient, that day, and that operation, I remain convinced that it was because I was so upset that I made the error that led to that complication.

Does your doctor drink? I noticed that I was getting a large number of patient referrals from the owner of a restaurant I frequented. I was puzzled by this since I could recall nothing that I had done to have warranted the owner's confidence in me as a physician. After the fifth or sixth referral, I asked what it was that had resulted in the restaurant owner's approval. "You are the only doctor who comes into the place and never drinks" was the reply. My abstinence was of value to them.

I must admit that since I view doing surgery as akin to an athletic event, I have been struck by the need to stay in good physical condition. This requires a degree of self-discipline that the patient should expect to see demonstrated in someone who is going to take them to an operating room.

Most of the questions, even "personal" ones, that I have been asked by my patients have been reasonable and appropriate. In truth, during my career in the practice of a surgical specialty, having taken literally thousands of patients to the operating room, I have been surprised at how few questions are asked by those who are about to undergo major surgery. They often preface their concerns with, "I know this is stupid, Doctor, but . . ." There are no stupid questions. I encourage you not to hesitate to ask questions of your doctor. Don't be shy. You do not need to be deferential. It is, after all, your body, and what is done to it—what you allow to have done to it—is, should be, and must be your decision.

Who Does What in the OR?

I can't tell you how many times a patient has said, "You are going to do the operation, aren't you, Dr. Barron?" It is true that most operations are done with one and at times two or more assistants. And surgical assistants do perform some aspects of the procedure. But how much they are allowed to do is up to the surgeon.

In teaching hospitals, an attending surgeon who doesn't allow the resident assistant the opportunity to do much of the case runs the great and, at times, significant risk of being unpopular. If you are to be operated on at a teaching hospital, put your wishes with regard to who your primary surgeon will be on the consent form. This is covered with a simple written declaration. "I am giving Dr. Warren permission to perform this operation." This will keep you from being operated on by assistants.

I have played the role of medical ombudsman to a prominent politician for the past twenty years. Not long ago he developed an irregular heart rhythm that required the placement of a heart pacemaker. When I left the operating room, it was my understanding that the attending cardiac surgeon would do the procedure. It was not until the operation had been completed that I learned that the surgeon had relinquished his role to his junior, a fellow in cardiac surgery. The procedure was being carried out while the patient was awake. He objected strenuously when he became aware of what was happening. After letting everyone in the room know in no uncertain terms that this was not acceptable, the primary surgeon stepped in and completed the procedure.

Since it is more than likely that you will be under general anesthesia and asleep during such a procedure, it is important that you make an official written record of your expectations on the operative permit that you and your surgeon will sign.

Second Opinions, New Technologies, Untested Skills

The difference between doing good and doing harm in medicine is finely balanced. Good surgeons, the famous saying goes, know how to operate, better surgeons know how and when to operate, and the best surgeons know how, when, and when not to operate. This is true for all of medicine.

As a result of medical insurance company policies, it has become common practice to obtain a second opinion prior to undergoing a surgical procedure. There are still many patients who elect not to follow this protocol. I believe this is a mistake. As a result of increasing medical technology, there are now many options that are appropriate in the management of the most common problems.

If you are going to have your gallbladder removed, it can

be done by the standard open technique or by laparoscopy, which has come to be known as the "Band-Aid" method. It was only after many complications, including deaths of patients undergoing this so-called minimally invasive surgical technique, that a consensus panel was convened and the conclusion reached that "the single most important variable that determines the safety and efficacy of laparoscopic cholecystectomy is the skill and . . . experience of the surgeon." New York State mandated that a surgeon must perform fifteen laparoscopic cholecystectomies under supervision before he or she would be eligible for independent operating privileges. I know that for some doctors five or six is an adequate number while others still don't get it right after doing five or six hundred. The importance of volume of a physician's experience has been acknowledged by many professional societies. For example, one of these groups reported that almost one third of hospitals that are approved to carry out open-heart surgery in 1994–95 performed fewer than two hundred procedures, which is the recommended minimum number for any institution. The idiosyncratic nature of medical practice as a function of experience is underlined by the data for Medicare beneficiaries. The proportion of women who have mastectomies rather than breast-conserving surgery for breast cancer in different regions of this country varies by a factor of thirty-five. This is attributable to the experience and practices of the physicians in the area where they receive their care.

Perhaps the most dramatic example of the role of experience is seen in the repair of an inguinal hernia, a defect in the muscles of the lower abdominal wall that results in a bulging out of the contents of the abdominal cavity. Every surgeon has been trained to repair this kind of hernia. And every surgeon who does the operation has a failure rate,

where the defect recurs. In good hands, this rate can be in the range of 5 to 10 percent. There is a hospital in Canada where they do this operation and nothing else. The surgeons who work there do more than six hundred cases apiece a year. This is more than most surgeons do in a working lifetime. They take less time, have the lowest failure rates, in the range of 1 percent, and charge less than in almost every other hospital. There is one caveat to this apparent endorsement. The surgeons who work at this institution have developed this expertise by being solely focused on the repair of an inguinal hernia. Some patients with an inguinal hernia may have other significant medical problems that fall outside the field of vision of such experts. If you are in the hands of such a technical wiz, you want to make absolutely sure that you have someone with a wider medical horizon looking over their shoulders. This person is commonly your PCP or the hospitalist. You must have detailed and specific discussions with this physician about all your relevant medical conditions that in all likelihood will not appear on the radar screen of the super-specialist.

There are many examples of this kind of super-specialization; just two are cataract surgery with the placement of an intraocular lens and joint replacement. If the super-specialist you have identified is not a participant in your plan, although it may require some negotiation, it is likely that your managed care organization will ultimately agree to allow you to have this physician perform the procedure at the MCO's standard fee. As to whether this super-doc will accept that amount as payment in full, you can negotiate that matter with him or her.

It is a difficult task for a doctor to reconcile the desire to learn a new technique with the knowledge that someone more experienced would probably do a better job with less potential risk to the patient.

The fifth article for the Declaration of the Informed Medical Consumer is: "Before I allow a physician to perform a procedure on me, I must know how many times the doctor has done this procedure, how frequently he or she does it, and how the patients have fared."

If a physician has done a procedure only a few times and relatively infrequently, you would be well advised to review your options with one who is more experienced and has a larger volume of patients who require the procedure. The question of a doctor's results is pivotal. Without knowing the details of how their patients have fared, you cannot possibly make an informed decision about whether you are willing to expose yourself to the risks of the procedure, of putting yourself in the hands of any physician.

This is especially important when you are going to have a procedure that involves a newly introduced technology or instrumentation. Patients prefer what has come to be known as "Band-Aid" surgery since such minimally invasive procedures have many potential advantages. They involve smaller incisions, smaller scars, and potentially shorter recovery times than standard surgical techniques. The major technical problem with this surgical approach is that it permits minimal access to internal organs, requires the use of instruments that are at best awkward to handle, and is usually performed using a miniature camera that projects the operative field onto a television screen. If this sounds complicated, it is! Someone has likened performing this kind of surgery to trying to tie your shoelaces using long-handled pliers while looking in a mirror. With that analogy in mind, you certainly want to know exactly how many times your surgeon has done such a procedure before you sign the operative consent form. In my experience, it is very unlikely

that a doctor will feel comfortable performing a technically difficult procedure until he or she has done it more than twenty or thirty times. And the dead last thing you need or want is an uncomfortable surgeon.

Minimally invasive surgical technology has been employed in such diverse situations as performing a hysterectomy, hernia repair, colon cancer, and even heart surgery. Surgeons naturally are encouraged to acquire the skills they need to perform these newly developed operations. Pressure from hospitals, equipment manufacturers, insurance carriers, and most important from patients leads to an increased demand for these new approaches. This demand very frequently outstrips the profession's ability to demonstrate that these new methods of treatment are both effective and safe.

When laparoscopic technology was first introduced to remove the gallbladder, the complications included everything from the inadvertent injury to vital organs near the gallbladder to patients dying during or after the operation. The use of the laparoscope in performing a hysterectomy, which is rapidly becoming a widespread procedure, has been associated with an alarming complication rate that is, in part, due to lengthy operating times with the associated risks of prolonged anesthesia and increased chance of infection.

Early in an individual practitioner's development of a skill, the potential benefits may be far outweighed by the potential harm that is a result of inexperience. The learning curve for some individuals may be steeper than for others, and while it should be incumbent on a surgeon to discuss his or her experience and level of skill with the patient, in my experience, I have not heard many physicians admit to their patients, while getting them to sign an informed consent, "By the way, this is only the third time I have ever done this procedure."

I believe it is because of the increasing complexity of options that it's vital to obtain more than one opinion. You need to ask yourself, Am I being given a recommendation that is the best one for me, or am I being driven by the physician's abilities and skills?

The additional motivation behind seeking and obtaining a second opinion, if additional motivation is necessary, is that the first opinion may just be wrong. Doctors are not infallible. While patients want to think that the critical decisions that determine the management of their illness are based on rigorous data, the decisions many physicians make are based on subjective clinical judgment. Not infrequently, these are not issues whose answers are simply right and wrong. You may find that one physician's judgment and explanation of his or her approach to your problem is more reasonable than another's. This is not an inappropriate basis on which to make a choice. Finally, if in the process of finding the right physician, you are faced with two who have the same opinion, it is incumbent upon you to choose the better of the two to perform the procedure.

I was recently given the assignment of counseling a patient with multiple myeloma. This frequently fatal cancer responded to the initial treatment and the patient became a candidate for a stem cell transplant. He was being cared for at a major university teaching hospital in New York City. However, when it came time for him to undergo this highly technical procedure, which can itself be fatal, we learned that although this institution had done many stem cell transplants in patients with other forms of cancer, they had only done one in a patient with multiple myeloma. Although we spent a great deal of time discussing the patient's options, it was a no-brainer, and he decided to travel to a major cancer center in Boston where they had greater experience with patients with multiple myeloma. When presented with the data, this decision was approved by the medical director for policy of his managed care company.

For many procedures, specialty organizations and medical societies have set a minimum number of a given procedure that a physician must do annually in order to maintain proficiency. For example, for the relatively new but increasingly performed procedure coronary angioplasty, the American Heart Association and the American College of Cardiology recommend that cardiologists who perform these procedures should do *at least* seventy-five angioplasties a year. If this were a regulation that was strictly enforced, it would mean that many cardiologists would have to stop doing the procedure. If you become a candidate for angioplasty, it is clearly appropriate for you to inquire about the caseload and experience of the invasive cardiologist that you will use. If his or her experience falls below these unofficial standards, you should request a referral to a physician and unit that meets or exceeds these numbers. Use the standards to make your case to your MCO.

The differences in the performance of this procedure and the consequences for the patients are startling. As many as 6.8 percent of patients whose doctors don't perform this surgery very often and who worked in hospitals where it was performed infrequently suffered complications that led to an emergency coronary artery bypass procedure or, worse, to death in the hospital. This is compared with a 4.6 percent complication rate when patients were cared for in hospitals with high patient volume where the physician caseload exceeded the standard of seventy-five angioplasties a year. For the Medicare population, this 2.2 percent difference translates into more than twelve hundred Medicare patients a year suffering adverse outcomes as a result of being cared for by a doctor with limited experience. Another study of this procedure provides graphic evidence that the best results are obtained by doctors who do at least twice the minimum number of angioplasties a year. The truth is that were 150 cases a year made the standard, only 5 percent of cardiologists would be approved and certified as being competent to do this procedure.

The bottom line is that the patients who get the best results undergo the procedure in high-volume institutions where the surgery is done by cardiovascular surgeons with large caseloads and experience. Remember, "minimally invasive direct vision coronary artery bypass" is in its infancy. There is very limited available data on this procedure, which is performed by few surgeons in very few hospitals but which may, in fact, be suitable for a large number of patients who are not now having it.

There is general agreement about the marked differences in outcomes correlated to experience of the operator with regard to newly introduced procedures. Since most will be done in a teaching hospital setting, it is vital that you be fully informed of just who is going to do what to you. You should know the name and rank of everyone involved in your care. While your own physician may be directing your care, many times it is the doctors-in-training who are designated to execute his or her instructions.

It is unreasonable for you to expect your doctor to return to the hospital at three o'clock in the morning to restart an intravenous line that has stopped working. On the other hand, if the individual who comes to reinsert a needle in your vein has failed after more than two attempts, and you learn that he or she is a third-year medical student, you are not being rude—in fact, you're being foolish—if you don't ask for a more senior member of the team. This isn't a trivial issue; there is a significant risk of bloodstream infection in patients who have intravenous lines in place. It has been estimated that more than 400,000 such vascular catheter-related bloodstream infections occur every year in America. The risk of these at times life-threatening infections is directly correlated to the method of placement of the line. Meticulous sterile technique is required in order to minimize the risk of infection. This includes the use of antimicrobial solutions at the skin site prior to the placement of the catheter as well as the application of a topical antibiotic at the point where the catheter enters the skin before the placement of a sterile covering bandage.

Procedures—Identification and Management of Risks

The physician in charge of your care has the responsibility to see that nothing involving your care is delegated to anyone who is not well qualified. It is your obligation to be vigilant to ensure that this is the case.

Procedures Where Experience Can Make a Big Difference

- All cardiac procedures
- All laparoscopic, Band-Aid, keyhole surgery
- All cancer surgery
- All vaginal surgical procedures
- All procedures to correct urinary incontinence
- All vascular surgical procedures
- All joint replacement surgery
- All neurosurgical procedures

Although for many procedures there is no recommended minimum number of cases that must be done for an institution or physician to be certified by the relevant credentialing body, the volume of cases for a particular operation done at an institution is available for the asking. If you want to know exactly how many hip replacements were done at your hospital last year, call the department of orthopedic surgery. The chairman's secretary can tell you where to get that information. You can find out the cesarean section rate in your hospital from the chairman of the department of obstetrics. In many cases, the interpretation of these data and how they should be used in your decision-making process requires the guidance of your primary care physician. But there is no question that you must know if your surgeon has done twenty or two hundred laparoscopic procedures. Present this information to your managed care organization when you are in the process of finding the right provider with the appropriate experience.

These are not theoretical issues, since new technologies are being introduced into the practice of medicine at a dizzying pace. There are significant financial forces that encourage the incorporation of these new methods and, at times, the use of almost experimental medications and procedures. Many times these demands outstrip the profession's ability to demonstrate the safety and effectiveness of new procedures through rigorous clinical trials.

Physicians try to balance their professional need for continued learning with the recognition that their income will be negatively affected if they do not incorporate the latest treatment methods in their practices, whether they are new operative techniques or new medications. Acquisition of the requisite knowledge and skill involves a learning curve. For surgical procedures, this curve is marked by complications that can be significant. Operating times for new procedures are always longer and involve being under anesthesia longer. As the surgeon becomes better and the OR team more familiar with the procedure, complication rates decrease as does operating time. While there is a natural tendency for the physician not to discuss these issues, you must explore in detail the surgeon's experience and his or her level of skill openly as a part of your decision-making process. This conversation must include not only the abilities of the surgeon and the others who will participate in the procedure but also possible complications, how they will be handled, and by whom.

The recent *New York Times* front-page story about the death of a thirty-one-year-old woman undergoing an elective procedure at a major teaching hospital in New York is a horrifying example of the results of inexperienced physicians using new high-tech equipment with an untrained support staff. A $30,000 fine was imposed on the hospital by the state regulatory agency after it was determined that the institution was culpable in the patient's death. In this case, it was reported that not only were the doctors who performed the operation not credentialed for that procedure, but as a result of previous poor performance they had been placed on probation by the director of their department, a disciplinary action that limited their independent privileges. The responsibility for the unnecessary, premature death of this young woman has to be shared by the managed care organization who, it is clear, made no effort to remove from their list of providers a physician whose professional performance was, at best, questionable. The salesman who represented the manufacturer that was trying to sell the new equipment to the hospital was in the operating room and involved in its operation during the procedure. Another very questionable practice! Regrettably, it is not rare for a physician to bring a patient to the operating room and plan to use

a piece of equipment for which he or she was essentially untrained in a hospital where the risk management program
did not automatically prohibit such behavior. In this case it
was reported the entire operating room staff, including the
nurses and anesthesia team, participated, apparently without significant objection.

The detailed newspaper and television reports about
this event made it abundantly clear that there were multiple
significant flaws in the process that would leave patients vul-
nerable. While you might reasonably expect that the checks
and balances to ensure patient safety would have come into
play, this did not happen. This unfortunate story highlights
the questions that you must ask when you are considering
undergoing any procedure.

You have to ask your physician the same questions
about newly introduced medicines: "How many patients
have you put on this medication, and for how long?" (Remember the recent debacle with phen-fen used as an appetite suppressant!) "How have they done, and what kind of
complications have you seen?" (Think about Seldane!)
When a newly introduced medication is prescribed for you,
you run the risk of complications that may be very severe
and even lethal. As the system of health care delivery becomes more complex and remote, only your vigilance will
protect you from taking unacceptable risks.

Informed Consent

Unless you're in a true medical emergency, a physician
must obtain your consent prior to rendering any treatment,
including performing an operation, carrying out many diagnostic procedures, administering anesthesia, or prescribing
a new medication or one with potentially serious side ef-

fects. Without such permission, the physician may be held liable for violation of your patient's rights regardless of whether the treatment was appropriate, rendered with the standard level of care, and has a positive outcome. A physician who provides you with medical care without such consent can be charged with "battery."

Informed consent is a process. It is often equated with the document that you are required to sign before the physician undertakes your treatment. In fact, this consent form is simply a legal document that certifies that there has been an exchange of information between you and your physician that has resulted in your accepting a specific treatment.

The active participation of both patient and physician is central to the completion of the consent form. As the patient, you are obligated to provide complete and accurate information and to ask questions to clarify any issues you don't fully understand. Your physician must provide you with all the information relevant to your ability to give a valid informed consent. There are many ways that this information can be provided, but the physician is obligated to allow you reasonable time to review all the information and encourage your questions in order to ensure that you fully understand the information. He or she is obligated to review all medically appropriate treatment options regardless of their cost or the extent to which the treatment options are covered by your health insurance plan.

The laws covering informed consent vary from state to state. Most states make this a responsibility that the physician cannot delegate to anyone else. There are two standards that are most usually used for determining if the informed consent process has been properly carried out. The "reasonable physician" standard is measured by what is customary practice in the medical community for physicians to divulge to patients. The "reasonable patient" standard has become of late the appropriate operating principle for informed consent. In this case, the question to be answered is, Has the patient been given the information that a reasonable person in the patient's position would want to know under similar circumstances? This standard is based on the patient's perception rather than on the doctor's perception of what the patient should be told.

This is not a trivial difference, since as a rule the professional or reasonable physician standard almost uniformly requires that less information be given than is the case where the reasonable patient standard is employed. If a risk of a procedure is highly unlikely but can have serious consequences for the patient, this information would have to be disclosed under the reasonable patient standard but could be omitted if the reasonable physician standard was being followed. As a practical example, consider that *every single operation* carried out with the use of anesthesia has death as a possible risk. While it is rare, there are patients who suffer an irreversible injury from the use of an anesthetic, and go on to die without any surgical procedure having been done. For example, patients who are improperly intubated by the anesthesiologist can suffer irreversible brain damage as a result of having an inadequate airway. While this rarely happens, a physician must discuss this kind of complication so the patient can provide a truly informed consent.

At a minimum, your doctor must discuss with you the diagnosis and nature of your illness, the nature and purpose of the treatment, the risks and potential complications that are associated with the treatment being recommended, the reasonable alternative treatments with the risks and potential complications associated with each alternative, the definition of a successful outcome, the relative probability of success if the treatment is undertaken, and finally, the predictable result if you choose not to be treated. Consent is "fully informed" only when you understand all of this information. There is no informed consent if the treatment extends beyond the scope of the consent.

In genuine emergencies, the process of informed consent is not in force. Special informed consent rules apply when the patient is a minor unless the patient is "emancipated" by virtue of living apart from his or her parents, is self-supporting, married, in the military, or, in the case of women, are demonstrably sexually emancipated. This permits minors to obtain treatments related to sexual activity, such as contraception, pregnancy, and sexually transmitted diseases. As with all patients, it is the physician's responsibility to see that the minor is fully informed before any treatment is given. If the minor is not emancipated, except in emergencies, the consent must be obtained from the patient's parent or legal guardian.

CHAPTER 5

Complementary and/or Alternative Medicine

While "health care" has become a politically correct phrase, the fact is that physicians are not trained to take care of the healthy. Precious little time in medical school and residency training is devoted to the healthy person or preventive medicine. Doctors are trained to care for the sick, to diagnose and treat disease. The standards of care for conventional medicine are those that have been proven safe and efficacious through an orderly process of animal testing, statistical analysis of controlled clinical trials, and published peer-reviewed studies. Treatments that do not have this kind of scientific basis are a part of what has come to be known as complementary or alternative medicine. These nonconventional therapies are widely used and deserve a review to determine which are useful, which are useless, and why. It is very important, before you embark on one of these treatments, for you to understand what we know and what we don't know about them.

You might think that simple, well-described, common diseases are easily diagnosed. Regrettably, in many cases, this is not true. These are the patients physicians describe as "interesting." Listen carefully when you are in the elevator in a hospital—this is the term you will hear when one doctor is talking to another about a patient with an as yet undiagnosed problem. Another term you will frequently hear is "difficult." This is often reserved for patients who have not responded to treatment.

It can and does happen that, even after impeccable effort on the part of excellent physicians, the patient remains undiagnosed. Some diseases are just very difficult to diagnose. The patient's symptoms may be transient, some may be very vague or difficult to describe. Some patients will have a common disease but its manifestations may mislead the diagnosing physician. Some diseases are rare; others are new. Think how long it took between the description of the first patients with symptoms of AIDS until it was accurately described. The same could be said for many other infectious and sexually transmitted diseases first seen in large numbers of patients in the past twenty years. Lyme disease is another example. Some diseases are chronic and run a slow, indolent course that compromises their ready identification.

When patients remain undiagnosed, they are usually besieged by well-meaning friends and family with advice. This most often includes the use of nonconventional approaches: "Take vitamin E!" "Take vitamin C!" "Take zinc!" "See my chiropractor!" There is, I believe, only one reasonable approach when you don't feel well and after all your efforts you have received no useful advice from your physician: You need a second opinion.

Many doctors who fail to identify what ails you recommend waiting for some period of time—days, weeks, perhaps months—to see what happens in the hope that the illness is self-limiting and will resolve itself without ever being identified or treated. This suggestion is colloquially known as "tincture of time" and is often made in hopes that the disease will identify itself with more classic manifestations. This is easy for the doctor to say, but it may be hard for you to accept. I have reluctantly come to the conclusion that this strategy is employed far more frequently because the physician's ego gets in the way; he or she is unwilling to admit that the problem might be solved by someone else with a fresh approach or more experience.

This having been said, the undiagnosed patient should be comforted by the physician who says, "I would like to get some help on this." Absent the physician making this recommendation, it is perfectly acceptable for it to come from the patient. No reasonable doctor would be offended by the undiagnosed patient who wants an additional review by another physician.

There is one significant pitfall to following this route. The second physician might be very tempted to be less than thorough in his or her review as a result of the biased assumption that if another "good" physician didn't find anything, there may not be anything there. It is not only possible but also likely that a second physician will not make a diagnosis when that has been the outcome of the first thorough workup. This may not be a reflection of inadequacy on the part of either physician. Medical knowledge is incomplete. Many questions don't have answers.

Standard or conventional treatment refers to mainstream medical treatments that have been tested following a strict set of principles and proven to be both effective and safe. Only after the results of such clinical trials have been reviewed and approved by the Food and Drug Administration can a treatment be considered a standard of care. Investigational treatments are those currently under evaluation. Alternative therapy refers to treatments that are unproven because they have not been scientifically tested or have failed to pass the rigorous testing required by convention. When such methods are used, the patient may suffer from the lack of treatment by standard accepted methods or because the alternative treatment is itself harmful. The term *complementary treatment* is usually reserved for those treatments that are used in addition to mainstream medical methods in order to relieve symptoms. Stress management, therapeutic massage, acupuncture, and biofeedback are examples of modalities that are employed not necessarily to cure a disease but simply to modify its manifestations.

More than one third of the adults in this country have used at least one unconventional form of health care during the past year. In a variety of surveys, 60 percent of physicians recommended alternative therapies to their patients at least once a year. Forty-seven percent of these doctors admitted to using such therapies themselves, and half that number have incorporated them into their medical practices.

The factors that have proved to be instrumental in patients choosing these nonmainstream approaches include a distrust of conventional physicians and hospitals, a desire for control over their own health matters, dissatisfaction with conventional practices, and belief in the importance of one's inner life and experiences, which are thought to be ignored or discounted by conventional medical practitioners. When questioned about their decision, patients most frequently offer one of two views: "I get relief for my symptoms/The pain or discomfort is less or goes away/I feel better," or "The treatment works better for my problem than standard medicine." Since the vast majority of medical symptoms are self-diagnosed and self-treated, it is important that the implications of this behavior be understood.

Evidenced-Based Medicine

The foundation of traditional medicine in America rests on what has recently come to be described as evidenced-based data. The pivotal questions about the value and risks of any treatment of a disease are answered by what are called random-controlled clinical trials (RCTs). The RCT is an experiment where patients with a disease are randomly allocated to one of the treatments or interventions under study and their response to this treatment is measured. The responses of all the patients in one treatment group are contrasted with those in the other. These data are subjected to a statistical analysis and a conclusion reached about whether one treatment is in a rigorously defined way "better" than another. These experiments can be very complicated and expensive, and can involve a large number of patients, doctors, and institutions. The patients in each treatment group may have to be matched for those traits that are important in the natural history of the disease under study—for example, age, gender, duration of illness, and the like—before being randomly assigned to one treatment or the other. More than two alternative treatments may be included in a single clinical trial. The trial may be what is known as a "blind" study, where the patients—and, in a double-blind study, the doctors evaluating the response being measured—do not know what treatment they are receiving. Although randomized trials work well for drugs, it is harder to test other types of treatments with them. There are many, many medical innovations that have been embraced without any demonstrable proof of their efficacy or safety, let alone a precise definition of their benefits or risks. The use of diethylstilbestrol (DES) to prevent spontaneous abortions, which not only didn't work but caused severe problems in the offspring of mothers who took this medication, and the use of radiation for the treatment of minor skin conditions such as acne are two examples of the unwise widespread use of risky treatments. Assertions, speculation, and testimonials are the basis for much support of such arguments that there are too many, as well as too few, cesarean section deliveries or open-heart surgical procedures today. These cannot and do not substitute for accurate scientific evidence. Consider the following example. Endarterectomy. The carotid artery is one of the main supply routes of blood to the brain. When this blood vessel becomes narrowed, there is an increased risk of stroke. A carotid endarterectomy is a surgical procedure to correct this problem. Since its introduction more than forty years ago, it has been very controversial. This operation requires exceptional surgical skill, and in the best of hands is associated with significant risks. In the past fifteen years, there has been a dramatic fall and a subsequent rise in the rates of carotid endarterectomy as a result of the publication of unfavorable reports that were followed by favorable ones. In 1988, a study showed that almost one third of the operations were done without the appropriate indications. Subsequently, very specific guidelines have been established with respect to the condition of the patients who would benefit from this procedure and the centers where the surgery should be performed. Regrettably, there is substantial data that these have been ignored to the detriment of many patients. The recognition of these practices should prompt you to ask questions when any new therapy or invasive procedure is recommended by your physician.

Without the kind of data that is generated in statistically valid, controlled clinical trials, any conclusions about the advantages or risks of the treatment of a disease become nothing more than anecdotal and therefore cannot be presented as proof of the efficacy of the treatment under consideration. It is the issues of a rigorous proof of efficacy and safety that are at the heart of the questions physicians have concerning the use of alternative medical strategies in any illness.

Historically, unconventional medical care was thought to be the exclusive domain of the charlatan. As a result of tabloid, radio talk show, and television news reporting by nonphysicians with the title "doctor," there has been an incredible proliferation of new and untested approaches to the maintenance of health and the treatment of disease. Many of these have found their way into the most prestigious of academic medical centers absent any critical evaluation. In large part, for political reasons, alternative medicine has recently been given a free ride. There should not be two kinds of medicine. We must rigorously test what we do and underwrite that which is proven to be safe and effective.

Alternative and complementary techniques often emphasize the relationship between mind, body, and spirit. Many focus on the internal and external causes of dysfunctions rather than responding to the patient's diagnosis or manifestations of disease.

When treating patients with incurable and/or chronic diseases, most physicians take no issue with the use of treatment methods of unproven value that have been shown to have a minimal risk of significant adverse effects. When caring for patients with fatal illnesses for which there is no chance for cure, any reasonable physician will accept the decision by a patient to choose an alternative medical therapy. In fact, as many as 60 percent of patients with cancer seek some complementary or alternative medical intervention during the course of their disease. Almost half of the physicians caring for these patients admit to giving them from tacit approval to outright encouragement.

The understandable dilemma for the traditionally trained physician arises when the patient considers these questionable methods in other situations. This has become a more and more frequently encountered challenge for practicing physicians. It has been estimated that there are 425 million alternative practitioner visits in the United States each year. This is 40 million more visits than were made to primary care physicians in 1997. It is striking that of the almost $14 billion spent on alternative medical interventions, more than $10 billion were unreimbursed expenses that were out-of-pocket payments for the patient. There are more than 300 different treatments and techniques that can be a part of complementary or alternative medicine. The main therapies include exercise, prayer, relaxation techniques, chiropractic, massage, diet, nutrition, bioelectromagnetic devices, and pharmacological and biological treatments including herbal medicines. The traditional medical practices of China, India, Tibet, and other cultures are a part of this group of therapeutic approaches. Some of these alternative techniques have been incorporated by conventional physicians.

Acupuncture, which is now widely used by physicians involved in pain management, is still considered by many to be of debatable use in many situations. Although there have been many clinical studies of its potential utility, most of these have generated equivocal results. It has, for example, been shown to be no more effective than a placebo in smoking cessation or weight loss. However, promising results have been reported that demonstrate the efficacy of acupuncture in the control of nausea and vomiting in postoperative patients and with cancer patients receiving chemotherapy. There is an enormous body of anecdotal evidence about its utility in the treatment of neck pain, headache, osteoarthritis, rheumatoid arthritis, asthma, and stroke; however, the rigorous examination of the currently available data does not support any such claims.

Allergies, arthritis, hypertension, digestive diseases, anxiety, and depression are all conditions for which conventional medical interventions have mixed results or are associated with significant adverse side effects. The widespread popularity of alternative medical approaches to these conditions is a testament to the failing of conventional therapies, *not* a rigorous demonstration of alternative medicine's efficacy.

A fundamental tenet of medicine is *primum non nocere*—the first thing (is) to do no harm. The lack of scientific proof for most alternative methods should sound an alert when proven effective treatments for a disease exist and are readily available. If a proven therapy exists, withholding that treatment would at the very least be harmful. If the alternative therapy has the potential for significant adverse effects whether proven or not, this can represent a potential for harm. If the alternative has no downside and there is no recognized effective conventional treatment, then it may be used with impunity.

The failure to generate the data necessary to be assured that a treatment is safe and effective is even more glaring in the existing evaluation of many widely used alternative medical therapies. An Office of Alternative Medicine has been established at the National Institutes of Health to coordinate as well as support and conduct research in alternative and complementary medicine. Public demand has also resulted in some health insurance companies reimbursing charges associated with some alternative therapies. If such treatment is covered by your managed care plan, you should not view it as definitive evidence that the treatment is either effective or safe. While physicians, insurance plans, medical centers, and policy makers should base decisions regarding the incorporation of and payment for medical therapies on evidence-based research and cost-effective analyses, in fact, consumer interest, market demand, competition, medical reports, and political pressure from well-organized groups with a specific agenda often drive the process. This is problematic for patients regardless of whether the treatment is a conventional or alternative medical regimen.

The majority of physicians have a great deal of difficulty accepting any nonconventional treatment protocols. This frequently manifests itself as anger or hostility. Patients often respond to their physicians' undisguised disapproval by seeing an alternative practitioner without telling them. This results in patients often being secretive about treatments they are being given and/or pharmacologically active substances they are taking. This puts you at risk. You must tell your physician about any alternative treatment you're having.

The aggressive marketing of common herbs for the treatment of such diverse symptoms as anxiety, constipation, depression, fatigue, insomnia, memory loss, tension, nausea, and fluid retention; and conditions such as alcohol abuse, arthritis, high blood pressure, high blood cholesterol, hemorrhoids, menstrual irregularities, enlarged prostate, stomach ulcers, urinary tract problems, and varicose veins—all of which can be associated with serious but treatable diseases—are dangerous. In view of the fact that none of the herbal remedies for these conditions has been subjected to controlled clinical testing, it is very important that they be used only after it is clear that these symptoms don't hide an underlying condition that requires treatment to avoid potentially serious medical problems.

Consider the herbal extract St. John's wort, which is being taken by many individuals for the treatment of depression. Available in health food and vitamin stores, the extract contains many pharmacologically active substances. The key ingredient is thought to be hypericin. The concentration of this substance in the commercially available preparations of St. John's wort is very, very variable. While studies have been reported that have mixed results, no RCTs have been published in this country that compare the efficacy of St. John's wort with that of the standard doses of the standard drugs used for the treatment of depression. Since St. John's wort is considered a dietary supplement by the FDA, it is not required to undergo the rigorous testing and close scrutiny of a prescription drug. With the variability of the concentration of active ingredients and the potency, purity, and safety of the various formulations of this and other herbal medicines largely unknown, you should understand that the risks may be considerable.

Sources of Information

From the reports you hear from various sources—radio, television, newspapers and magazines, books, the internet—alternative medicine doesn't always adhere to the basic medical tenet "first, do no harm," and many, if not most, fall far short. This is probably accurately attributed to the conflict between goals that are often on a collision course. These stories are often presented by news reporters who are journalistic generalists and have no expertise in medicine or science. They often rely on an expert who may or may not have been directly involved in producing the new finding. In a story that may take two minutes of airtime or be confined to five hundred words, there is a simplified presentation that does not include the appropriate frame of reference in terms of the risks of treatment, alternative approaches, or available data on the outcome of the "newly" discovered therapy. After hearing these reports, patients often come to the doctor thinking they have the disease of the day and can be cured by the end of the day.

Judging whether the information is applicable and creditable is a greater challenge than finding it. The internet is a rapidly accessible data source for patients, relatives, and close friends to get information on serious and potentially life-threatening diseases. It will provide electronic mailing lists, on-line support groups, and web sites devoted to the particular disease. Information on the web can give you a sense of control and improve your ability to participate in decisions about your health care. This may even improve your sense of empowerment at a time when illness has undermined it. However, you will have little ability to determine how reliable this information is.

There are now literally hundreds of sites on the web that focus on alternative approaches for a variety of diagnoses. I have taken the opportunity to sample just a few. The following are potentially valuable resources that I found easy to use:

- The Center for Complementary and Alternative Medicine, maintained by the University of California at Davis, is primarily focused on the treatment of asthma and allergies with acupuncture and herbal therapy.
  http://www-camra.usdavis.edu/
- Fact Sheets on Alternative Medicine, maintained by the Columbia Presbyterian Medical Center, include a variety of data resources and information on alternative therapies.
  http://cpmcnet.columbia.edu/dept/rosenthal/factsheets.html

- The FDA Guide to Choosing Medical Treatments outlines the criteria that are employed in evaluating the safety and efficacy of new treatments together with information concerning current clinical trials of alternative treatments. *http://www.fda.gov//oash/aids.fdaguide.html*
- Phytochemical and Ethnobotanical Databases, which deal with information about medicinal plants, have been established by the Southwest School of Botanical Medicine. *http://www.ars-grin.gov/duke/*
- U.S. National Institutes of Health, Office of Alternative Medicine, maintains a web site on alternative medicine. *http://altmed.od.nih.gov/*
- The University of Texas Center for Alternative Medicine Research is dedicated to studying the effectiveness of complementary and alternative therapies used in the treatment of cancer. *http://www.sph.uth.tmc.edu/utcam/default.htm*

The *Journal of the American Medical Association* has a "Patient Page" that presents information in a consumer-oriented style. These pages are available as a free service from the AMA. The page includes a "for more information" section with toll-free numbers and web sites for governmental as well as nongovernmental agencies that have material relevant to the subject. The goal of this project is to provide the public with unbiased effective and reliable information about significant medical problems. They have included a discussion of alternative and complementary medicine approaches in a variety of diseases.

In view of the uncontrolled growth of health information on the internet, most of which has not been validated by accepted methods of peer review and evaluation, there are real questions as to whether it is possible to put this information to such a test. Much of this information is produced and exchanged by groups of people with common interests and views. Evaluating subjective, context-dependent criteria is difficult at best.

The widespread recognition of the potential for quackery among cyberdocs has led to the development of internet web sites that are devoted to calling attention to such activities.

QuackWatch, *www.quackwatch.com,* developed by a retired psychiatrist, includes hundreds of products, services, theories, and advertisements that can charitably be characterized as misleading.

The U.S. National Council Against Health Fraud, *www.ncahf.org,* is another registry of subjects and organizations it considers of questionable practice.

With this in mind, admitting my biases, I strongly urge the following cautions before you turn to alternative medicine:

- Don't treat a symptom without knowing its cause.
- Don't stop taking prescribed medications without first speaking with your physician.
- Tell any complementary practitioner about any medications you are taking.
- Tell your doctor about any complementary or alternative treatments you are receiving.
- If you are pregnant, trying to conceive, or breast-feeding, do not take any herbal medicines.
- If any symptoms persist or worsen during alternative therapy, consult a physician.

CHAPTER 6

Major Medical Concerns: Pay Attention and Sweat the Details with Your Managed Care Organization

Y ou are most likely to have a conflict with your managed care organization when you have an important medical problem. It is when you are fully occupied with the concerns of your disease that you will have to take the initiative to make sure you have the right doctor, the best hospital, and the right treatment.

In the past, when there were few or no choices in the management of a problem, it took very little time for a physician to review treatment options with a patient and his or her family. This is no longer the case. And now, high-technology therapies have assumed a starting role even for such comparatively straightforward conditions as pregnancy. You should remember that every time a new technology is introduced, there is the inevitable time lag before a managed care organization will include it in its contracts with enrollees. An example of the problem of having care covered by an MCO can be seen when one considers the care of patients with heart disease. Twenty-five years ago, someone with chest pain attributable to coronary artery disease would undergo angiography and a decision would be made concerning the patient's suitability as a candidate for bypass surgery. If suitable, the patient was taken to the operating room in short order and underwent the required surgery. Today, that same patient with the same history has a confusing variety of options, some of which are considered experimental by many managed care companies and are therefore not routinely covered.

This is also true for many cancers. Today, a man with prostate cancer will, depending upon his age, be offered a number of different treatment approaches. These will include radical surgery, several different forms of radiation therapy, hormonal medications, and sometimes even just watchful waiting. In the case of breast cancer, new interventions of unproven value include bone marrow or stem cell transplantation.

It is because of this variety of choices in treatment that your approach to your managed care organization must be proactive. This is the only way for you to ensure that you don't confuse your options or limit your choice of treatment as a result of your MCO's policies with regard to whether they will pay for a specific treatment.

Pregnancy and Maternity Care

There are more than 4 million hospital admissions annually in the United States for obstetrical care. More that one half of these women will have a normal vaginal delivery. It is only as a result of the professionalization of obstetrics that a normal biological event has been co-opted and redefined as requiring hospitalization and the attention associated with such institutionalized care.

I have often characterized the practice of obstetrics as 99 percent boredom and 1 percent stark terror. Over the past fifteen years, the proportion of women who have received care early in their pregnancy and had the recommended number of prenatal visits to their doctor has increased. In addition, there is evidence that during this same period a significant number of women have received more than the recommended amount of care. Yet, the signal indices of prematurity and low birthweight have not improved during this same period.

In fact, for women who are having a normal pregnancy, any invasive intervention must be questioned. This is not to say that prenatal screening based on blood tests is unreasonable. However, the definition of which women are at high risk of having an abnormal baby is a moving target that has been revised many times during the past twenty-five years. This is not because there has been a change in the risk of having an abnormal baby or that some previously unrecognized risk has been uncovered. Amniocentesis and chorionic villus sampling, invasive screening procedures that can detect some fetal abnormalities—procedures that are not without risk of injury to the mother and baby—have been applied to more and more women. This has happened as the age of the mother at which such procedures are recommended has dropped steadily over the past twenty years. There are several reports that support the conclusion that these changes have in part been based on the desire to reduce the likelihood of a malpractice suit that almost inevitably follows the delivery of an abnormal baby. This is not the only instance in obstetrical practice where legal, not medical, considerations have prevailed in the decision to implement a specific program or intervention.

We have mounted major efforts for the detection of rare events with little or no examination of the relative costs of such screening programs. The use of fetal monitoring of 100 percent of women in labor has become the accepted target for hospitals without a critical appraisal of its cost or benefits. Over the past twenty-five years, the rules for intervention in pregnancy and labor have been written, rewritten, and revised again with little or no rigorous examination of the effects of such changes.

While there are questions about the application of these screening tests, you should make sure that your physician explains your options and understands your wishes. There should be no question about your coverage for these services and/or associated genetic counseling. If there are any issues in this regard, they should be resolved with your managed care organization using the strategies discussed in Chapter 1.

A significant number of women who expect to have a normal spontaneous vaginal delivery have decided that traditional hospital care is unnecessarily intrusive. Many of these women have elected to have their maternity care provided by a nurse-midwife and/or to deliver at a free-standing birthing center. Many hospitals have created birthing rooms and hospital-based birthing centers in response to the needs and demands of these women. In my opinion, it is only this group of otherwise healthy women with no other medical problems, such as diabetes or high blood pressure, who can with a high degree of safety receive their maternity care from a certified nurse-midwife with oversight by an obstetrician who can intervene if and when that should become necessary. This model for the care of the pregnant woman is as, if not more, desirable than the standard level of obstetrical care that is delivered routinely in hospitals. However, you should determine your MCO's policies with regard to coverage for these services. Many available maternity care options are not covered by every managed care company. Since these practices differ from one organization to another, you should determine your MCO's policies and negotiate a resolution for any issues with regard to coverage. Although you may be required to obtain medical clearance from an obstetrician, you can be assured that if you elect to use such an alternative to routine obstetrical care, you can prevail with you managed care organization.

There is real doubt and legitimate debate about the high-tech interventions that are routinely employed in the labor and delivery suite in the hospital, and whether they have resulted in a measurable improvement in the outcome of the birthing process in healthy pregnant women going through a normal labor that will end with a spontaneous vaginal delivery. In women who have no problems that could complicate their pregnancy, it is commonly recommended that they see their doctor once a month until the twenty-eighth week, and then every two weeks until the thirty-sixth week, and weekly thereafter until delivery. These guidelines were developed after it was shown that such surveillance permits the early identification of correctable conditions that, if not treated, can lead to significant problems for both the mother and baby.

However, the questions that women should repeatedly ask their obstetricians throughout their pregnancy include:

- Is my pregnancy following a normal pattern?
- Is the baby the right size for this stage of my pregnancy? If not, is the baby too small or too large?
- Do you think I will have any problem delivering vaginally?

The use of ultrasound during pregnancy has provided the expecting mother with a picture of her developing baby in the womb and the obstetrician with a precise view of the developing fetus so that these questions can be answered with some degree of reliability. Only if your pregnancy is progressing normally is it appropriate for you to consider alternatives to standard in-hospital delivery.

If you choose a nonconventional option, you must be sure that you'll be able to transfer rapidly into a conventional obstetrical care setting if complications develop. You must review this contingency with a case manager and understand the managed care organization's policies before you elect nonroutine obstetrical care. Because of complex issues with regard to the reimbursement for professional services—who gets paid for what during the nine-month course of a pregnancy and the delivery—there may be restrictions to your coverage that would lead to your choosing a more traditional form of maternity care.

Another very important issue in deciding who will provide maternity care has to do with the manner in which the majority of obstetrical and nurse-midwife practices are organized. These providers are, in the main, now practicing in groups. This means that if your obstetrician is in a group that has a "one in five" schedule for night and weekend coverage, there is only a one in five, or 20 percent, chance that you will be delivered by your regular doctor or nurse-midwife if you go into labor at night or on a Saturday or Sunday. With this organizational structure, it is very important for you to become familiar with all of your maternity care provider's associates, since you won't know which one will be in charge of your care during your labor and delivery. You must also be assured that all the providers who cross-cover for your obstetrician or nurse-midwife are certified participants in your managed care organization.

*   *   *

There are many information resources for the pregnant woman. Several of them are sponsored by nonprofit organizations with a record of making substantial contributions to the care of pregnant women. These include the March of Dimes Resource Center, (888) 663-4637; National Maternal and Child Health Clearinghouse, (703) 356-1964 or *nmchc@cirsol.comwww.cirsol.com/mch;* and the American College of Obstetricians and Gynecologists, *www.acog.org.*

If your pregnancy is considered high risk, you have very different concerns. Regardless of the basis on which this conclusion is reached, whether it is your age, the presence of an abnormality during the pregnancy, the history of a significant medical problem such as diabetes or high blood pressure, or a prior pregnancy that was marked by a complication in the mother or infant, you should, if at all possible, be evaluated and, if necessary, managed by an obstetrician who specializes in high-risk pregnancy. Certification in maternal and fetal medicine is the credential that validates an obstetrician's training in the delivery of care to such high-risk patients. There is no question that if you fulfill the clinical criteria for a high-risk pregnancy that your MCO will provide coverage for such a super-specialist, though there may be some questions, on the margin, about whether or not you fulfill the definition. This is one of those issues that you may have to bring to a case manager. However, you should be aware that there is no question, if you are indeed at high risk, that your obstetrician will strongly support your being approved by the MCO for this care. This is one issue that has already been tested in court.

There is substantial data that physicians with this training are best prepared to provide care to high-risk women. Since it is the maternal-fetal medicine specialist who will make the critical decisions as to how and when screening for a genetic defect should be performed, or if the baby should be delivered by an elective cesarean section, there should be no question that this is the routine practice under any managed care program.

Regardless of whether your pregnancy is considered normal or high risk, it is important for you to take a pro-active role in your maternity care. This is true if for no other reason than the enormous increase in the proportion of babies delivered by cesarean during the past twenty years. Cesareans have historically been associated with higher professional fees and hospital charges. Managed care organizations have decreased the differential between the reimbursements for a routine vaginal delivery and a cesarean. It is not that MCOs have created guidelines that interfere with the obstetrician's decision, but they have stopped rewarding the doctor who charges higher fees for sections.

Hospitals and health plans are often ranked on the basis of cesarean delivery rates, with the implicit assumption that lower rates reflect more appropriate, more efficient clinical practice. However, this is a complex issue, since cesarean delivery is clinically indicated in many situations. Maternal age, breech presentation, fetal distress, history of a prior cesarean delivery, and many other patient-specific factors are appropriately a part of the decision-making process. Although there are large differences among hospitals, practices, and providers with regard to the proportion of babies delivered by cesarean, these differences are difficult to interpret, and each individual case deserves a detailed discussion with your physician.

Because of the wide array of choices, you should review all the inclusions and exclusions of any managed care plan with respect to maternity care before you select it. Even the most restrictive of managed care plans has some options with regard to the choice of a provider. Prenatal care that includes birthing and Lamaze classes may or may not be covered under a given plan, and many plans cover care provided by nurse-midwives. While many exclude the cost of obstetrical delivery in a free-standing birthing center, they will pay for care if the facility is within a hospital. Most MCOs explain that this decision is based on the safety of having the hospital-based obstetrical services readily available in case a problem arises that cannot be adequately managed in the free-standing birthing center.

Investigate the cesarean rate of both your physician and the hospital where you expect to deliver. There are large differences in these rates among doctors and institutions. Debate continues about the indications for a cesarean delivery, but it is appropriate to review your physician's approach early in the pregnancy. Since questions have been raised about the once-inviolate rule "once a cesarean, always a cesarean!," this discussion is justified even if you have had one in a previous pregnancy. Because of the way many obstetrical practices are organized, it is necessary for you to cover this topic with each of the physicians who might attend your delivery. In part because their providers cannot perform operative obstetrics, women who receive their maternity care from nurse-midwives are far less likely to have cesareans than women whose care is provided by an obstetrician. There is an inherent bias in this observation since the patients who have sought out obstetricians for care or cannot be cared for by nurse-midwives have problems associated with an increased risk of requiring a cesarean. In any event, it is a good idea to have a detailed discussion with your doctor in the early stages of your pregnancy about all of the aspects of labor and delivery.

Infertility Treatments

The coverage of the treatment of infertility under managed care is more variable, more inconsistently provided, and more frequently revised than almost any other medical condition. If this becomes a problem for you, without doubt, you will have to deal with the managed care organization, recognizing that regardless of their apparent contractual commitment, their practices truly are implemented on a case-by-case basis.

Whenever the apparent capriciousness of their policies with regard to the treatment of infertility is challenged, the claim is made that it is as a result of the incredible pace of the introduction of new and innovative technologies. There is no doubt that assisted reproductive techniques (ARTs) have brought about a revolution in the treatment of infertility. These technologies include a variety of procedures. In vitro fertilization (IVF) involves hormonal treatment of the woman in order to maximize the production of mature eggs in a given cycle. The eggs are surgically removed from the ovary and mixed with sperm in the laboratory. After about forty hours, fertilized eggs are subsequently placed in the uterus. Approximately 75 percent of ART cycles use IVF, with a 20 to 25 percent success rate. Gamete intrafallopian transfer (GIFT) involves the placement of eggs and sperm into the fallopian tube with fertilization occurring there. It is used in approximately 5 percent of cases with a success rate of around 25 percent at good centers. Zygote intrafallopian transfer (ZIFT) uses eggs that are retrieved after hormonal stimulation, fertilized with sperm in the laboratory, and then injected into the fallopian tube. Currently, two percent of ART cycles are ZIFT, with a success rate that is approximately the same as GIFT.

While the introduction of any new drug is preceded by

a long process involving the expenditure of large sums of money, which is rigorously regulated by the government, there is no such oversight for the introduction of assisted reproductive techniques. According to the Society for Assisted Reproductive Technology, the success rate for deliveries per egg retrieval procedure was 22.5 percent of 41,087 cycles of IVF attempted in 1995. That is up from 20.7 percent in 1994. In 1995, in the United States, 11,631 women gave birth to 16,520 babies as a result of assisted reproductive technologies, with large differences in the results of the various methods from one center to another.

One cycle of IVF can cost as much as $8,000 to $10,000! Since many couples have to undergo more than one treatment, the costs of ART can be very high indeed. This makes the chance of success an important element in your decision about whether you are willing to shoulder these expenses out-of-pocket. The differentials in success rates are dependent on many variables, including the prospective mother's age and medical status. Women over age forty have a significantly lower success rate using their own eggs. They are more likely to have a miscarriage or give birth to a baby with a significant birth defect. These risks are substantially reduced if the older woman uses an egg donated by a younger woman.

The methods employed in the treatment of the infertile couple are changing at a dizzying pace, and it is not possible to predict what new approach will be used in the treatment of this problem even a month from now. But several caveats must be considered in any treatment of infertility. First, what are the success rates for a given technique at a specific center? Success is defined as the delivery of a healthy infant. It is not the number of eggs harvested from the woman who has undergone hormonal stimulation of her ovaries. It is not the number of eggs that have been fertilized using in vitro techniques. It is not the number of fertilized embryos that have been implanted in a woman's uterus. It is not the number of women who have had a positive pregnancy test. It is not even the number of pregnancies. It is the number of healthy babies taken home at the end of a hopefully normal pregnancy. It is clear that at this point, at most centers, few couples are voluntarily told of the relatively small chance of success.

It is very important for anyone embarking on the use of ART for the treatment of infertility to understand just how "experimental" these processes are at present. There is, for example, general acceptance that hormonal stimulation of the ovary is associated with a measurable increase in the risk of subsequent ovarian cancer. Also, a significant risk of ART that has been given very little attention is that associated with multiple births. There is substantial evidence that the woman and babies in multiple birth gestations are subjected to potentially severe complications and increased mortality. The relative risk of infant death for twins is 6.6 and for triplets 15.9 times what it is for single births. The risks to babies of multiple gestations include prematurity and growth and developmental abnormalities such as mental retardation and blindness. The risk of cerebral palsy is significantly increased among multiple births even when the infants have a normal weight at birth. There is no data that supports the conclusion that this group is also at greater risk of developing seizure disorders including epilepsy.

While there is the possibility of what is euphemistically called fetal reduction—a method of decreasing the number of fetuses that the mother is carrying—this is viewed by many as a form of abortion and may not be an option for some couples. Because of the recognized high risk associated with triplets and higher-order multiple births, researchers are investigating new techniques that will reduce the likelihood of IVF multiple births. You should discuss whether your doctor is familiar with these new methods.

Currently, the most high-tech of these interventions is intracytoplasmic sperm injection (ICSI). This involves the placement of a single sperm into an egg in a test tube. If fertilization is successful, the resulting viable embryo is placed in the uterus. This method is of use for those men with a low sperm count. Used in about 10 percent of cases, its success rate is not significantly different from GIFT or ZIFT. ICSI has been introduced and widely applied even in the face of some data that suggests that it is associated with the potential for chromosomal injuries that could result in significant genetic damage to the fetus. It is a technique that involves the physical manipulation of all the critical genetic apparatus of the potential baby. No extensive trials of the procedure, examination of outcomes, or risks of the process to the fetus have been carried out. Thousands of children have been born as a result of the use of ICSI.

While most of the published reports about ICSI have been reassuring, one study suggests that live infants conceived using ICSI appear to be twice as likely to have a major birth defect and nearly 50 percent more likely to have a minor defect than infants conceived using other in vitro methods. An even more troubling finding has been presented that raises the issue that ICSI-conceived children may have subtle and long-term deficits. These include both mental and psychomotor developmental defects. These same issues and questions must be raised with regard to many of the processes that have been incorporated in ART, such as the freezing and storing of embryos for varying periods of time prior to their implantation in a woman's uterus.

In addition to your questions about the cost and success rates of any procedure in patients of your age with your

reproductive history at the center where you are considering being treated, it is vital that you have a *full* discussion of
all the possible risks of the recommended treatment for the
mother, the father, and, if the procedure is successful, the
baby. Today, in the ART arena, you cannot simply assume
that what the doctor is recommending has been proven to
be both effective and safe.

The rapid advances in ART are driven by scientific discovery as well as by profit and patient demands. This is why
new techniques are adopted without rigorous studies to
demonstrate effectiveness and safety. For these reasons,
many managed care organizations have decided to exclude
ART from their covered benefits. So, you should exercise
caution before embracing any new ART method.

The resources for the infertile couple include Resolve,
a nonprofit support group, (617) 623-0744 and (888) 299-
1565 or *www.resolve.org*. Information on assisted repro-
duction is also available through the Centers for Disease
Control and Prevention, (770) 488-5706 or *www.cdc.gov/
nccdphp/drh/arts/index/htm*, and the American Society for
Reproductive Medicine, (205) 978-5000 or *www.asrm.com*.
Each of these organizations has an established record of
maintaining a substantive database. While there may be a
slight tilt to the material presented as a function of their
mandate, I have found them to be accessible and relatively
complete and accurate.

All of the revolutionary approaches to the treatment of
the infertile couple are extremely expensive, and the majority of managed care organizations cover only a very small
portion of the costs. You must review your contract with the
managed care plan very carefully to learn under which circumstances coverage is provided and the limits of that coverage. Since many if not most health insurance plans have

some limitations if not outright restrictions on ART procedures, you may find even after an extensive appeals process that your coverage for any of these ARTs is inadequate. It is very important for you to recognize that while you may not have insurance coverage through your MCO, the experts in this field are aggressively marketing their very lucrative services. If, after your appeals, the plan provides no or limited coverage for care of infertility, it may be appropriate to discuss a negotiated rate with your infertility specialist. Many reproductive medicine centers have entered into contractual agreements to provide their services at a discounted rate with one or more managed care organizations or other insurance carriers, so there is a negotiable fee schedule for the treatment of infertility. In discussing the cost of ART with a physician, you should ask about the fee he or she accepts under existing contracts with MCOs. This figure should be the basis for negotiating a fee that you can reasonably expect to have to pay. The medications that are used in the treatment of infertility are expensive. So you should explore with your managed care company the possibility of purchasing these drugs through their contracted suppliers. If you are able to get these drugs at a discount, you will want to separate the cost of medication out of your negotiation.

You should not be shy about dealing with the cost of this care. The treatment of infertility has been identified as a "cash cow" by both doctors and hospitals, which is why they are advertised so widely. There is a lot of room between the cost of providing these services and the customary charges quoted for both the physician and the facility. If you require treatment for infertility, I urge you to expend the effort to find the right provider at the right price.

Stroke

A stroke is the effect of damage to the brain that is caused by interference in its blood supply as a result of the blockage of a blood vessel, thrombosis, or a break in a blood vessel in the brain that leads to a cerebral hemorrhage. Approximately 80 percent of strokes are due to a clot in an artery in the brain; 20 percent are due to bleeding into the brain.

Although stroke has long been recognized as a leading cause of death and disability, it was recognized recently that the incidence of stroke has, in fact, been startlingly higher than was previously estimated. More than 700,000 Americans suffer a stroke each year; one third of them die as a result. Since the incidence rates will inevitably rise as the population ages, it is very important to recognize the symptoms associated with stroke and understand that there are significant benefits to prompt treatment. New drugs to dissolve blood clots materially affect the consequences of a stroke. Even if you only suspect that you or someone you know has had a stroke, call 911; consider it a medical emergency.

The warning signs of a stroke are:

- Sudden severe headache with no known cause
- Unexplained dizziness, unsteadiness, a sudden fall
- Sudden loss or change in vision in one eye
- Sudden difficulty speaking or understanding speech
- Sudden weakness or numbness of the face, arm, leg, or one side of the body

The factors that are associated with an increased risk of stroke are:

- High blood pressure
- Smoking
- Heart disease
- Diabetes
- A history of transient ischemic attacks (TIAs)

There have also been reports showing an association between stroke and a low level of a variety of vitamins as well as such infections as recurrent bronchitis and chronic periodontal disease.

The cornerstone of programs for the prevention of stroke are primarily behavior modifications. If you smoke you should stop; if you drink alcohol, it should be in moderation; if you are overweight, go on a sensible diet; if you have high blood pressure, diabetes, or high cholesterol, make sure that your physician has you on the best regimen for their control; and finally, stay calm. There is substantial evidence that men who experience outbursts of anger have twice the risk of stroke as those who control their tempers.

Rehabilitation becomes the central issue for stroke survivors. How well you'll do afterward strongly depends on starting and maintaining a rehabilitation program—and the sooner the better.

There are several reliable sources of information about stroke. These include the American Heart Association Stroke Connection "warmline," (800) 553-6321 or *www.amhrt.org;* the National Institute of Neurological Disorders and Stroke, (800) 352-9424 or *www.ninds.nih.gov.;* and the National Stroke Association, (800) STROKES or *www.stroke.org.*

The initiation of aggressive treatment of patients who suffer a stroke can result in a major difference in the eventual outcome. As with most true medical emergencies, when you are treated and who treats you are the crucial elements that determine the incidence of long-term complications and the likelihood of death. Since most people have little warning before a stroke, you should take steps to identify a first-class medical resource before such an untoward event occurs.

You should read your managed care contract to find out what care is covered and where that care can be provided. Regrettably, many policies do not adequately cover the costs of rehabilitation after stroke (or for that matter following a hip replacement or heart attack). This is another reason for knowing all the details of your health insurance contract and understanding exactly what coverage you have before you ever need any medical care. However, as with almost every condition but most especially in such areas as rehabilitation for a chronic condition, what is covered by the managed care company is dependent on the vigilance and initiative of your physician, who is, in fact, your chief medical ombuds- man. I have become involved in disputes about the provi- sion of this care for patients with a variety of conditions. It is sad but true that, as with almost every such interaction with a managed care company, at best, this becomes a semi- adversarial contest of wills. Unless you are extraordinarily well informed and aggressive, once again you will only pre- vail with the strong support of your physician, who can knowledgeably argue your medical need for rehabilitative services.

Cancer

There are more than 1.2 million new cases and more than half a million deaths from cancer in the United States annually. Beyond 2000, there will be a significant increase in the number of cancer cases as the baby-boom generation begins to reach the ages where the age-specific rates of certain cancers start to rise.

The most common cancers are lung, colon, prostate, and breast. With the exception of lung cancer in women, which is on the rise, the death rates from these malignant diseases appear to be leveling off and may be declining as a result of the detection of earlier, more readily curable, disease. Cancer is the leading cause of death for women between the ages of thirty-five and seventy-five. In this group, breast and lung cancer account for the vast majority of these deaths.

Today, while the sessions devoted to molecular biology at medical meetings are the most exciting and well attended, the fact is that gene therapy is still experimental. The clinical management of patients with cancer is and for the near future will be based on surgery, radiation therapy, and chemo and hormonal therapy. Surgery and radiotherapy are effective in many cases in curing localized disease. For patients whose disease has spread, radiation is used to control the disease locally while chemotherapy is used for systemic or distant disease.

Although substantial, the achievements of these conventional therapies have not fulfilled the many promises that have been made. While it is not unreasonable to expect that existing methods of treating cancer will soon be replaced by some major therapeutic breakthrough or advance in molecular biology, in fact, all reports in the press to the contrary, the major advances in the battle with cancer, to date, can be attributed to prevention and the detection of the disease at its early, curable stage.

Cancer Screening

There is widespread agreement that screening is justified for many cancers. For each malignancy, there are legitimate ongoing debates about exactly who should be included in a screening program. These arguments are based on many issues, including the cost of the test, the likelihood of an individual developing the cancer, and the risks of the screening test.

For example, we know that smoking is the overwhelming risk factor for lung cancer. There is no substantial data that screening for lung cancer among those not at high risk for this disease—nonsmokers—is a rational use of public health funds. There is also no question that screening all women over the age of fifteen for cervical cancer is beneficial. Taking a Pap smear involves no risk to the woman. The test is relatively inexpensive. And the benefit of detecting early cancer and lesions that are precursors of cervical cancer and 100 percent curable has been well demonstrated. There are, however, some questions as to how frequently the Pap test should be done. The differences are based on what are the known risk factors for cervical cancer.

There are far more complex issues with regard to screening for breast cancer. Risk assessment for this kind of cancer is very complex and more than three out of four women who develop it have no identifiable risk characteristics. Aside from age, which is a risk factor common to all malignant diseases in adults, a family history with a first-degree relative (mother, sister, or daughter) who is premenopausal with breast cancer is associated with a three- to fourfold increase in risk compared to women without such a family history. If more than one first-degree relative had breast cancer, the risk may be as high as eight to ten times that of the general population. Approximately 10 percent of women who are treated for breast cancer will develop a second primary cancer during their lifetime. A woman who has had no children or who has had her first full-term pregnancy after the age of thirty-five has an increased risk of this disease compared to women who had their children earlier in their reproductive life. Other documented risk factors for breast cancer include early age at first menstruation (before age twelve) and late age at menopause (older than fifty-three years of age). A prior history of malignant disease such as Hodgkin's lymphoma is also associated with an increased risk.

Recently, the medical reporter for one of the major television networks wrote a book with an extravagant title that claimed he had found a diet to prevent breast cancer. This medical celebrity hyperbole notwithstanding, there is no diet that has been proven to prevent any cancer. Many authorities cited the absence of data to support the assertion of the title. This is but one example of the hype that has invaded the presentation of almost all medical information presented in newspapers, magazines, and television. You must read and listen very carefully to these reports and the often exaggerated claims.

The American Cancer Society and the National Cancer Institute now recommend mammography annually for women without symptoms beginning at age forty regardless of risk. This recommendation is not supported uniformly, with some experts feeling that screening women under forty should be limited to those at risk for early-onset breast cancer as well as those with radiographically dense breasts for whom mammography is a relatively insensitive test. There is uniform agreement that women should have annual mammograms from age fifty to seventy-five. Randomized trials appear to show that screening mammographies can result in a reduction in breast cancer deaths by uncovering disease in women who are asymptomatic. The debates about the age at which such screening exams should begin, and the optimal time interval between successive exams, are based on population data with the analysis carried out to maximize benefits in the aggregate. These are very different issues from those focused on the advantages for the individual that can be gained by screening for otherwise undetectable disease. It appears that the benefit of breast self-examination in early detection has not been proven. This finding flies in the face of the almost uniform pressure on women by their gynecologists.

The complexity of breast cancer screening is demonstrated by the steps that are followed when a mammogram is not normal but not unequivocally diagnostic of cancer. If a mammogram documents the presence of a lump, an ultrasound examination is often performed to distinguish solid from cystic masses. It must be recognized that a normal mammogram at any age in a woman with a breast mass does not eliminate the need for further evaluation. The steps to be followed if a mammogram is abnormal may include other imaging techniques like magnetic resonance (MRI), computed tomograhy (CAT scan), or positron emission tomography (PET scan). Thermography has absolutely no place in the workup of a breast lump. Fine-needle aspiration (FNA) provides a sample of cells from the lump for evaluation under the microscope and can at the same time resolve any questions about a fluid-filled benign breast cyst. FNA does have limits, and even a negative result may not be definitive. Stereotactic biopsy is a newer technology that can confirm a diagnosis of cancer before an open surgical breast biopsy. Relatively few practitioners have the necessary skills for the use of this technique. The use of ultrasound guidance for needle biopsies of breast masses, which does not require expensive equipment, is currently gaining as the diagnostic method of choice. Ultimately, no mass can be completely assessed without a surgical specimen that can be examined under the microscope. An unequivocal diagnosis of cancer can only be made based on what is known as a tissue diagnosis.

The workup of a positive mammogram warrants a detailed discussion with your physician. There is no question that this is a situation that requires that you be comfortable with what he or she is recommending. Given that you agree with his or her recommendations, there should be no issue with regard to coverage by your managed care organization. If you do not agree, you will have to obtain a second opinion. This option is normally covered by MCOs either as a matter of policy or upon request through the utilization manager process.

In contrast, although some studies have suggested the potential advantages of increased detection of early stomach cancer, there has been no concomitant decrease in mortality from this disease. The most effective way to reduce deaths from stomach cancer will probably be through primary preventive measures including diet, vitamin supplements, antioxidants, and the elimination of *Helicobacter pylori,* the organism associated with stomach ulcers. There are data that support the utility of screening for colon cancer with three randomized trials having been carried out that showed a reduction in mortality among those who were detected with early disease.

The questions that are raised with regard to the testing for prostate cancer are complex. Currently, the issues in this regard deal with the costs associated with population screening. Although there is no data that can provide rigorous proof that lives will be saved by such screening, there are strong indications to support the conclusion that early detection and efficacious treatment could be effective. The naysayers in this argument point to the enthusiasm for lung cancer screening several years ago, which came to nothing. Again, these negative views are solely concerned with population data and how much it costs to find one patient with an asymptomatic cancer. While it should be understood that questions of the general public welfare and the optimal use of health care dollars are a significant part of discussions with regard to population screening for cancer, no one can sensibly argue against an individual electing to be screened for any potentially lethal cancer where the test itself is associated with no risk and the response to a false positive result, where the person is judged to have the disease and in fact the test result is wrong, also bears no possible adverse consequences.

Screening strategies for colon cancer are perhaps the best demonstration of the difference between individual benefits and the optimal allocation of health costs for the public in general. It has been claimed that periodic colonoscopy could reduce the risk of bowel cancer essentially to zero for all those without the genetic predisposition to developing this disease. This expensive and somewhat uncomfortable procedure has been adopted voluntarily by many on the recommendation of gastroenterologists who adhere to the widely accepted theory that this technique permits the detection and removal of those precancerous lesions that, if undetected, would go on to develop into invasive cancers. There is no doubt that, based on cost alone, routine screening colonoscopy cannot be justified on a public health basis. While there are many examples of the dichotomy between the individual and public good with regard to screening for disease, this example is one that has as its hallmark the individual's motivation to minimize the risk of developing colon cancer. In addition to screening, the best preventive actions include eating a diet high in fiber and low in fat, which appears to reduce the risk of developing bowel cancer.

All in the Family

The single factor that is associated with the most marked increase in risk of colon cancer seems to be a genetic disposition, which appears in families who demonstrate a high incidence of a variety of cancers. Families with this genetic constitution are now readily identifiable.

The media attention that has recently been focused on cancer genes has called attention to one's increased risk of developing a familial or heritable form of cancer. A cancer is considered to be heritable if it occurs in at least three individuals from at least two generations, and if at least one affected individual is a first-degree relative of the other two. Breast, ovarian, and colon cancers, to name just a few, have been associated with the presence of both familial and heritable forms of the disease. If you are a member of a cancer-prone family, you will need to consider intensive screening tests. There are risks, benefits, and limitations of such risk assessment screening tests, including the potential for loss of employment, insurability, and the health of your relationships and your outlook on life as a result of their outcome. If you have been identified as a member of a cancer-prone family, you and your physician will have to bring this matter to the attention of your managed care organization in order to be provided coverage to screen for the genes that have been associated with an increased risk of developing a cancer. In my own experience this coverage has never been disallowed by any managed care organization when the question has been raised.

Insurance Coverage for Cancer

With the continuous discovery and introduction of new methods for the treatment of almost all important cancers, it is practically inevitable that insurance carriers will view many of these new therapies as not medically indicated, investigational, or experimental—and therefore not covered. As with all other diseases that are likely to involve a very high financial cost, you should review the coverage provided by your plan before signing on.

The most frequently cited reasons for selecting a health care plan include best value, affordability, and ability to use a specific doctor in the plan. In fewer than one third of cases do enrollees in managed care plans even mention coverage as a factor in making their selection of a given plan. Since it is very difficult and requires a substantial effort to get any insurance carrier to extend care for anything not included under a specific contract, the first issue to be considered prior to choosing a plan is to fully understand the coverage that you are paying for and can get without question.

When an issue of coverage is raised it is vital that the professional providing the service be willing to be your active ally in dealing with the insurance carrier. If a participating physician—either the primary care doctor or the specialist—is not willing to join forces with you, you have a long uphill battle. In any event, the process of negotiation is the same whether this disease is cancer or any other illness (see Chapter 1). You must keep detailed records of all exchanges as you work through the bureaucracy of the insurance company. If you are unable to resolve that issue after you have discussed your case with the medical director in charge of clinical practice policy for the treatment of cancer, you will be forced to seek satisfaction outside the company. To briefly review your optimal strategy, you should consult other cancer specialists who can be cited as unquestioned experts. If the dispute cannot be resolved through medical venues, write to the governmental licensing agency of managed care organizations, which is commonly the state commissioner of insurance. When faced with your managed care company's persistent denial in spite of medical support with regard to the validity of the treatment for which coverage is being disallowed, seek out the support of your elected representatives in the local, state, and federal governments (see Chapter 1 for details).

Living with Cancer

As a result of our success in detecting and treating early disease, more and more people are living with cancer. There are a host of medical issues that these people must face, including a greater risk of infection as a result of both the disease and its treatments, radiation therapy, chemotherapy, and surgery. An additional and very significant side effect of these treatments is malnutrition, which can have devastating effects on quality of life and survival. Cancer-induced malnutrition is due to many factors, including loss of appetite, nausea, vomiting, and an altered sense of taste and smell. Depression and anxiety also contribute to decreased food intake. In combination, these can have major effects on food intake and the sensation of fullness.

Every individual undergoing treatment for cancer should also undergo a nutritional assessment. Not infrequently, newly diagnosed cancer patients have unintentionally lost 10 percent or more of their body weight in the previous six months, resulting in loss of muscle strength and depletion of fat stores. The goal of nutritional support for people living with cancer is to reverse or prevent such a deterioration of their general health. Some people may benefit from such strategies as eating several small meals and the use of commercially available high-calorie liquid nutritional supplements. It has been shown that just paying attention to the details of a person's food intake alone is often sufficient to achieve the goal of weight maintenance.

In my own practice, this has proven to be one distinguishing feature that has helped patients maintain a good quality to their lives for a protracted period of time even while going through treatment, or eventually succumbing to their disease. Recognizing that cancer chemotherapy destroys the appetite for many, if not most, patients, it becomes very important to pay meticulous attention to the nutritional value of foods. When patients identify the foods they like, they will eat those foods even when they are not hungry. Since taste and smell are affected by many of the commonly used anticancer treatments, many find that highly seasoned foods that they avoided in the past are now palatable, even tasty.

It is only through trial and error that you will find what foods are best for you and will help you maintain your weight. Since this is the measure of success, it is very important to confront reality and routinely weigh yourself every day. In order to succeed, it is necessary to pay the same fanatic attention to detail as someone who is dieting to lose weight. For this reason, in the same way that I monitor my patients who are overweight, I weigh my cancer patients at every follow-up visit and make a point of recording and discussing any change since their previous visit.

Preventing Cancer

Epidemiology provides compelling evidence that many cancers may be preventable. Tobacco use remains the largest single avoidable cause of premature death and the most important known carcinogen to man. Between 25 and 30 percent of all cancers among those in developed countries are tobacco-related. On the basis of thirty studies, the U.S. Environmental Protection Agency has concluded that environmental tobacco smoke—passive smoking—is a carcinogen to the human lung. It has been estimated that every year there are more than 400,000 deaths in the United States directly attributed to tobacco use, in particular cigarette smoking; 112,000 of these are due to lung cancer. Alcohol consumption is causally related to cancer of the mouth, larynx, and esophagus. The effect of alcohol appears to be enhanced by cigarette smoking. Exposure to sunlight increases the risk of developing skin cancer. There is accumulating evidence that certain viruses are associated with an increased risk of cancer.

There is some data that suggests that certain naturally occurring and pharmaceutical products have the potential to stimulate or prevent the development of malignancies. It appears that an increased intake of fat and red meat is associated with an increased risk of colorectal and probably prostate cancer. High consumption of fruits and vegetables is associated with a reduced risk of lung, pancreas, larynx, esophagus, bladder, and stomach cancers.

There are a vast number of studies now under way to evaluate the relationship between a variety of chemical agents including vitamin A in lung, mouth, and skin cancers; vitamin C in colon and stomach cancers; vitamins D and E in breast, skin, cervix, colon, lung, and stomach cancers; as well as such pharmaceutical agents as aspirin, antibiotics, hormones, and selenium in liver and lung cancers; calcium in esophagus, bladder, and colon cancers.

Perhaps the most dramatic recent report of a method to

prevent cancer has involved the use of a drug called tamoxifen for the prevention of breast cancer. The manufacturer has initiated a direct-to-consumer notification program explaining the risk of developing breast cancer and the information that their drug has been approved to reduce the occurrence of breast cancer among women at high risk of developing the disease. The campaign will include providing on request a free video that provides details to prospective users. Unfortunately, this drug appears to increase the risk of uterine cancer; blood clots in the arms, legs, and lungs; strokes; and the formation of cataracts.

Treating Cancer

The treatment options for individuals with cancer are changing at a dizzying pace. One typical example of the technological revolution in the treatment of brain cancer is the gamma knife. Originally termed *radiosurgery*—the delivery of high doses of radiation to a small target on a single exposure—this technique, used initially for the treatment of benign tumors and other nonlethal disorders in the brain, has recently been used for the treatment of brain cancers. Radiosurgery has become an adjunct to the standard interventions of surgery, radiotherapy, and chemotherapy for this group of tumors. Not every institution has a gamma knife or the staff with the necessary training or experience to use it.

Every day, new techniques or methods of management for the treatment of cancers are proposed or approved for trial. The customary method of reporting these findings has been a published report in a medical journal. In many cases, this has been replaced by an announcement on the national evening news programs. You must understand that these new methods of treatment have not yet stood the test of time. New medical treatments of all kinds should be viewed like new model cars. It takes a year or two before you know if there are going to be any significant recalls to repair manufacturing defects. No medical treatment is without risks. Although approval by regulatory agencies comes after safety and effectiveness have been demonstrated, these studies do not and cannot uncover infrequent events or events that occur after long-term exposure. Even very large clinical trials are inadequate to assess the potential of a treatment to induce a rare but serious side effect. Your managed care organization may not provide coverage for new treatments that require additional surveillance before being certified as safe. In addition, you should appreciate that initially the skills and knowledge to use any new treatment are limited to a very few physicians. It isn't until that experience becomes more broadly based that it is reasonable to expect that these technologies will be readily available or that your managed care organization will include them among the treatments for which they provide coverage.

There are literally tens of thousands of resources that can give you the latest information on cancer treatments. The National Cancer Institute (NCI), an arm of the National Institutes of Health, publishes a series of pamphlets that deal with prevention, detection, and patient education. The NCI's information service can be reached at (800) 4-CANCER. This is the basic, first-line resource for patients with cancer. The NCI also has a web site for health care professionals. Beyond such established organizations such as the National Cancer Institute and the American Cancer Society, web site resources of medical information must be reviewed with some caution. There is no way of knowing whether what is being presented is based on science or snake oil. It can be confusing and dangerous. There are any number of professional-looking sites that offer little more than anecdote, opinion, or inaccurate information. This is even more often true in the case of cancer.

The NCI is the best place to begin a search for almost any question concerning the diagnosis and treatment of any malignant disease. The NCI has created the world's largest database and communication structure dealing with all forms of cancer. This includes such technical information as the drugs of choice for the treatment of cancer as well as services for patients. There are several different entry points into this data. CancerNet, *hhtp://cancernet.nci.nih.gov,* is a web site that is produced jointly by several different government agencies. PDQ, *http://cancernet.nci.nih.gov/pdq.htm,* is the NCI's comprehensive, computerized cancer information database. It is a knowledge base detailing "original research papers, summaries on state-of-the-art treatment, supportive care, screening and investigational drugs" that is updated monthly. PDQ contains the most up-to-date information available about cancer prevention, early detection, and treatment that can be found on the net. Unlimited access to the PDQ file is available to the public at a modest cost. The NCI Cancer Information Service, *http://cancernet.nci.nih.gov/occdocs/cis/cis.html,* is a description of a free telephone service where patients and physicians alike can call to get information and directions from the nineteen regional offices of the NCI Cancer Information Service. This service will provide the answers to questions concerning treatment and care options for any type of cancer. The National Cancer Institute Cancer Centers Program, *http://cancernet.nci.nih.gov/global/glo pt.htm# nci-designated,* lists the e-mail addresses, telephone numbers, and web sites of NCI-designated cancer centers across the country. This is the entry point for those who are looking for the highest quality cancer care in their region. A collection of literature citations on seventy different topics is included in the National Library of Medicine's Cancerlit database, Cancerlit Topic Searches, *http://cancernet.nci.nih. gov/canlit/canlit.htm*. A typical entry will consist of the title, author, source, and abstract of a recently published article. The last six monthly editions of each topic are available at the web site.

There are several other oncology resources. OncoLink, located at the University of Pennsylvania, *http://oncolink. upenn.edu,* is designed for use by patients and physicians. This site includes data on the financial aspects of cancer care and has a very useful section on frequently asked questions. The American Cancer Society, *http://www cancer.org,* includes data on the most common cancers. This database has a substantial focus on patient education materials. CanSearch is a site that has been developed by the National Coalition for Cancer Survivorship, *http://www. access.digex.net/~mkragen/index.html*. This not-for-profit agency attempts to mobilize psychosocial resources for cancer patients and their families. This base includes a section on current clinical trials that would be of value to any patient newly diagnosed with cancer. Cancer Care, Inc., *http://www. cancercareinc.org,* is a site that is supported by grants from philanthropic organizations and individuals. It provides a range of services that includes patient counseling, social services, physician referrals, and financial assistance.

These resources are starting points for finding the information that is relevant to any form of cancer. There is no other disease for which there is such a wealth of well-organized information. However, even with all the available data, there are many unresolved issues and questions where you'll find incompatible answers given by experts with equivalent credentials. The treatment of breast cancer is, perhaps, more controversial than almost any other malignant disease. A large comprehensive study of current practices in the management of breast cancer suggests that tens of thousands of women are undergoing mastectomies and having their breasts removed unnecessarily. For the vast majority of the 180,000 women diagnosed with this disease, almost 75 percent are eligible for breast-conserving surgery, commonly known as a lumpectomy, followed by localized radiation therapy and possible subsequent chemo or hormonal therapy. Almost one in five women for whom a lumpectomy with follow-up treatment is appropriate elect to undergo a mastectomy. While there is still some disagreement as to whether this is the best treatment for women with "a bad breast cancer," it has been uniformly acknowledged that a mastectomy confers no advantage in terms of life expectancy for those without such an aggressive malignancy. An additional heated debate in the treatment of breast cancer involves the use of bone marrow or stem cell transplantation in association with high-dose chemotherapy.

These are examples of why it is so critical that you examine all treatment options and discuss the problem with several independent physicians. Only after this kind of review can you determine what treatment you should select and work through the process with your MCO that secures your chosen course of therapy.

As with any disease for which the answers provided by conventional medicine can range from cautionary to obscure, there is a strong tendency to reach out to alternative resources. There are a host of organizations that actively market to patients who have failed to respond to or suffered a recurrence of their cancer following conventional therapies. More than 50 percent of patients diagnosed with cancer will not be cured by the standard care regimens of NCI-certified cancer centers. So it is not surprising that there is a large demand for treatment modalities that have yet to be proven effective by well-designed and -executed clinical trials. As I think back over the time that I have been in practice and cared for patients who eventually died of the cancers that brought them to me, I am very hard pressed to be dismissive of any steps that they took outside of the conventional medical arena.

Jane O'Toole was a very healthy sixty-eight-year-old woman when she experienced the sudden onset of lower abdominal pain that she attributed to a "gas attack." After three similar episodes over the course of a month, she was diagnosed with pancreatic cancer that had spread to many of her internal organs, including her liver. In order to avoid a potential disaster as a result of what was clearly an imminent obstruction of her intestine by the tumor, her doctor recommended an operation. She agreed and went through the procedure. All this care had been provided at an NCI-established cancer center.

Her postoperative course was stormy and marked with several serious and frightening complications. When she had recovered, she convinced her doctor that she wanted to hear the unvarnished truth about her prognosis. It took substantial effort for both of them, but in the end it was clear that there was no hope of cure. The doctor did go to great pains to emphasize that regardless, she would be treated with what was currrently the favorite drug for pancreatic cancer. When she learned that he was convinced that this would result at best in a few additional weeks of life but was associated with some significant and unpleasant side effects, she asked for some time to think things over. For the next several weeks, beset by the inner turmoil of coming to terms with her imminent death and besieged by friends and family to get additional opinions, she went from doctor to doctor looking for a different view of her situation and some alternative to the recommended therapy. Once she came to terms with the fact that no reputable establishment physician involved in the care of terminally ill patients with cancer of the pancreas offered any other treatment program or outlook, she decided to turn to alternative resources. This was for her a frightening journey down a path that had been taken by hundreds of thousands, perhaps millions, of incurable cancer patients. She came to the conclusion that she would have to travel to Germany and undergo a series of treatments that involved a serum or vaccine prepared from her own blood and the subsequent repeated inoculation with that vaccine. She had been my patient for many years and came to see me.

As I had recognized so many times before, here was a woman with a terminal illness for which there was indeed no hope of cure. I could in good conscience, therefore, mount no significant objection to her seeking solace from some other quarter. While I had my doubts that this clearly experimental program would change her clinical course in any meaningful way, I was convinced that for her psyche this was the very best thing she could do.

Shortly after her visit to my office, Mrs. O'Toole left for Germany. As things turned out, several trips to Europe were required. Upon each return home, she came to see me. Finally, with the vaccine in hand, she asked that I continue to give her the required inoculations according to the schedule that had been prepared by the German physicians. To my great astonishment, in addition to her subjective report of generally feeling better since beginning the vaccine treatment, there were objective findings including a decrease in the size of the tumor masses in her liver as demonstrated on follow-up CAT scans.

Mrs. O'Toole lived in reasonably good spirits for more than a year before the disease broke out of whatever had held it in check. In all candor, this was far longer than any of us would have predicted at the time of her diagnosis. She came to see me just three weeks before she voluntarily entered a hospice. She was absolutely convinced that she had done the right thing and that she had lived as long as she had as a result of her foray into alternative medicine. Believing that regardless what path she chose, there would have been very little difference in the eventual outcome, I gained some comfort from knowing that she was at ease and had derived substantial satisfaction in maintaining her sovereignty and self-determination during the final stages of her life.

In taking care of the Mrs. O'Tooles in his or her practice, your physician should be supportive even when you choose to deviate from accepted conventional standard therapies. Yet it is possible that you might bring a request your physician cannot fulfill without some risk. When Mrs. O'Toole asked that I administer the vaccine that had been developed in Germany, it raised the issue of my taking part in an activity that could void my malpractice insurance coverage with respect to the care of this patient. I made the decision to accept the risk that the patient or a member of her family might initiate a suit in the future, since I thought this was a highly unlikely event. Since there is no way to guarantee that this will not happen and no way to indemnify the physician against such an untoward potentially personal costly event, a physician might choose not to agree to undertake this responsibility.

As with any chronic disease, it is absolutely vital if you have cancer that you establish and maintain a comfortable relationship with your physician. It is, however, even more

264 / Outsmarting Managed Care

critical that you be assured of the competence of your physician. It takes a very skilled team of doctors to care for this group of patients, and such a collection of specialists is usually only available at or working in association with a major academic medical center.

Heart Disease

The leading cause of death in the United States is heart disease. It is the number one killer of men over age thirty-five and the number two killer for women between thirty-five and seventy-four. Heart disease and associated complications account for almost a million deaths a year and is the number one killer in all developed countries. A heart attack is the most obvious sign of heart disease. Every year in the United States, 1.5 million people have a heart attack, and a third of them die within twenty days.

In no case does data exist that is more compelling in terms of revealing the difference in outcome for patients with heart disease who receive a high quality of care as contrasted with those who do not. Recently, a series of reports have recorded the startling differences between physicians with regard to their approach in the management of patients who have had heart attacks.

The largest of these studies considered the effects of peer review on the care of patients hospitalized as a result of a heart attack. A review of this report demonstrates that changes in the routine practices of physicians require enormous effort and support of respected clinicians who are widely accepted as expert and who, as a result, will be effective agents of change.

A family history of heart disease, being male, African American and over age sixty-five are risk factors for heart disease. And more than half a million women over sixty-five die from cardiovascular disease, primarily as a result of a heart attack. While most of this mortality is confined to women over the age of sixty-five, almost 20,000 women under that age die as a result of a heart attack every year. One third of these women are under the age of fifty-five. To put this in perspective, breast cancer kills 43,500 women a year and all cancers combined account for 250,000 deaths among women each year. The risk of heart attacks is lower in women than in men in middle age. Apart from hormone-related diseases specific to their sex and the enormous difference in the risk of ovarian as compared with testicular cancer, coronary heart disease is the most deadly disease showing a sex bias. Women's lower risk cannot be simply attributed to the use of hormone replacement therapy (HRT) among menopausal women. This does not argue against the benefits of HRT, for there appears to be significant positive effects among women who take this medication.

The end stage of heart disease is chronic heart failure, a common problem with a grim prognosis that affects 3.5 million people in the United States and is the only cardiovascular disease that is increasing in frequency. The 250,000 deaths and one million hospital admissions cost almost $40 billion a year. The ultimate treatment of these patients is heart transplantation, which, with current technology, roughly doubles the life expectancy of these patients. Expert medical management has greatly improved duration and the quality of life of patients with heart disease. Even interventions as simple as the addition of yoga-based breathing exercises has been shown to improve the well-being of patients with chronic heart failure.

Smoking, high cholesterol, heavy alcohol consumption (more than two drinks a day), excessive stress, high blood pressure, diabetes, obesity, a high-fat diet, and physical inactivity are all risk factors for heart disease that are under your control. For postmenopausal women, estrogen replacement therapy has been shown to reduce the risk of cardiovascular disease by as much as 50 percent.

A heart attack occurs when a blockage or obstruction in the coronary arteries that supply blood to the heart reduces or stops the flow of blood to the heart muscle. This will result in damage or death to a part of the heart muscle and is known as a myocardial infarction. The blockage of the blood flow can be caused by a blood clot (coronary occlusion or thrombosis), or by the growth of plaque on the inner lining of a coronary artery (a process called atherosclerosis).

The symptoms of a heart attack are sudden chest pain, ranging from a tight ache to severe crushing pain, commonly radiating to the shoulders, arms, neck, or jaw. The pain is not relieved by rest and is often associated with shortness of breath, sweating, nausea, and/or vomiting.

It is imperative that you recognize and immediately respond to the symptoms of a heart attack. Your treatment options depend on how much time elapses between the onset of symptoms and the initiation of treatment. New medications dissolve blood clots and such surgical interventions as coronary artery angioplasty can mechanically widen a narrowed coronary artery. These treatments work best if you get to the hospital within a few hours after the onset of symptoms. Plus, you need to be treated at a facility that has experience with the use of the new and very effective methods for treating this potentially life-threatening event. This is another compelling reason for you to research the most qualified hospital near you (see Chapter 3). Call 911, and chew an aspirin tablet while you're waiting for the ambulance.

James Dale, a physician, was visiting his sister at her home in Virginia when he experienced a bout of severe chest pain. He was slightly nauseated. He was only forty years old, and although a pack-a-day smoker, he had no other identifiable risks of heart disease. He attributed his symptoms to indigestion and didn't even report them to his wife for almost an hour and a half. By the early afternoon, when the pain was not relieved by an antacid, and knowing how all hospitals work, he decided to go to the hospital rather than wait until a later hour, when the daytime staff had left for the day.

Within an hour of arriving at the hospital, Dr. Dale was in the interventional radiology suite undergoing an angiogram. This X-ray identified the clot in his major coronary artery. An injection of one of the clot-dissolving substances did not work, but while he was on the X-ray table he received another drug and watched the monitor as the clot dissolved and blood once again flowed through the previously blocked artery.

Almost instantly, his pain resolved and as far as Dr. Dale was concerned, he was ready to leave the hospital. Everyone prevailed on him to stay through the night. By the next day, his electrocardiogram was absolutely normal and the blood tests that would have been expected to document damage to his heart muscle were also completely within the normal range. For all intents and purposes, this patient, who, without any doubt, had suffered a blood clot in his coronary artery, had sustained absolutely no demonstrable damage to his heart muscle—because he acted quickly and got to the hospital without delay.

So, understanding the symptoms of and treatment options for a heart attack maximizes the likelihood of securing the best available care.

The introduction of new technologies has had no greater impact on medical therapy than in the treatment of heart disease. Patients can be offered a menu of choices including closed procedures that require a minimum of surgery as well as a number of different open surgical procedures such as bypass done through a small incision in the chest wall with the surgery performed on a beating heart; this avoids the use of the bypass pump associated with a variety of potential intraoperative and postoperative complications. Most recently, the Food and Drug Administration has approved the use of a new technique known as laser transmyocardial revascularization. Its use is restricted to patients with severe coronary artery disease.

Which of these options you'll hear about and what suggestions will be made depend on your physician's training and experience. Since, for the vast majority of patients, any of these interventions can be scheduled electively, you should have time for a detailed examination of each option with several different physicians. Choose the one with the most technical expertise for the procedure.

This is another instance where you will want to carefully explore all your options. Your primary care physician will refer you to a cardiologist who has the mandate to instruct you about the spectrum of choices that are appropriate for you. After you have explored these alternatives and settled on one, you will enter into discussions with your managed care organization. As with all such highly specialized care, you will need your physician as a strong ally if it is necessary for you to go out of network. In the treatment of heart disease, you must ask questions about the necessity for any intervention. Every option has significant risks.

You should not assume that if the treatment you have selected is not approved by your managed care organization that the decision was made simply to save money. It is possible that they have come to a conclusion that the risk-benefit equation for the treatment is questionable and are waiting for additional data before providing coverage for it. An example of the need for caution in the area of newly introduced treatment methods is the recent debate over the use of lasers to create new blood vessels in the hearts of patients with severe angina. The immediate appeal of such a high-tech method attracted a lot of attention and proponents without adequate proof that the procedure had improved exercise capacity or survival. The initial wave of enthusiasm was based on reports of noncontrolled clinical trials; some of these had been partly funded or designed by the manufacturers of the laser equipment. These reports emphasized the relief of chest pain without demonstrating objective improvement. This has been followed by skepticism, and now pessimism, as the results of a large, well-designed controlled trial led to the conclusion that, at best, laser therapy was likely to be useful in a very limited group of patients. Until better knowledge of the effects of the laser beam, including damage to the heart, is known, this technique should be considered experimental. Furthermore, until that information has been collected, the technique should be used only in a research setting. This kind of information is considered by your managed care organization when making a decision about providing coverage and should be included in your discussion about these matters.

For more information about heart disease, the American Heart Association, (800) 242-8721 or *www.amhrt.org,* and the Information Center of the National Heart Lung and Blood Institute, (301) 252-1222 or *www.nhlbi.nih.gov/nhlbi/ nhlbi.htm,* are excellent, unbiased resources.

Diabetes

There has been a marked increase in the incidence of diabetes, which is one of the most common chronic diseases in the United States with a prevalence of almost 8 percent. Diabetes is associated with an increase in the risk of developing cardiovascular disease (CVD). It has been estimated that as much as 30 percent of all CVD occurs in people with diabetes and is the most common complication among people who are non-insulin-dependent diabetics. Cardiovascular disease probably accounts for 50 percent of all deaths in diabetics and cerebrovascular disease and stroke for another 15 percent. These rates are as much as twenty times those in similar adults who don't have diabetes. People with insulin-dependent diabetes are also at increased risk of CVD!

Prevention and intervention can do a lot to avoid CVD complications in diabetics. Since the risk factors for cardiovascular disease are well known, and can be present long before the clinical diagnosis of diabetes, it is important for anyone with these risk factors to be screened. Changing whatever risk factors you can is an important goal for the prevention of complications in diabetes.

If you have diabetes, you have to be very careful about diffuse injury to the small blood vessels in the body, which can lead to significant damage to the kidneys, eyes, and most probably the nerves. These complications are a result of a combination of metabolic, hormonal, and genetic factors. It appears that "tight control" of the disease through aggressive medical management can delay the onset and slow the progression of these aspects of the disease.

If you discover that you have high blood cholesterol, high blood pressure, or abnormalities of blood clotting mechanisms when you're first identified as diabetic, you'll need to have these problems treated aggressively to delay the progression of the most ominous complications of diabetes.

Vigilant medical attention has resulted in a lower incidence of such complications as blindness, end-stage kidney failure, limb amputation, and coronary heart disease. "Watch and wait" has absolutely no place in the treatment of anyone with diabetes.

More Than One Disease

Many people, especially those with a chronic disease, are more than likely to develop a second or even a third disease at some point. Regrettably, it is not uncommon that when one problem consumes the doctor's attention, the other disorders often escape detection and/or treatment.

So, women with diabetes are much more likely to develop coronary artery disease; they may also need hormone replacement therapy after menopause. People with emphysema or chronic lung disease are far more likely to be severely affected by a relatively minor cardiovascular insult. People with psychiatric illnesses such as depression frequently experience a worsening of their mental status when suffering a physical ailment. While this is a more common problem for senior citizens and the elderly, it is also a risk for younger patients. You and your doctor must be vigilant to be sure other problems aren't being overlooked.

Your Health Is in Your Hands

It is clear that your medical care will in very large measure be determined by the decisions of your employers. If they can provide this care in conjunction with workplace health initiatives and general wellness programs, which ultimately help the bottom line at a reasonable cost, they'll do it. Yet, nowhere is the value of prevention demonstrated more clearly than when considering the real costs of these programs. It is significant that unhealthy lifestyles cost

Americans an estimated $200 billion in health care expenses every year. Smoking, excessive drinking of alcohol, drug abuse, and unsafe driving are choices that put you at risk. If you want to improve the chances that your managed care company will have the money to increase your coverage, do what you can to remove these risks from your life.

INDEX

About the Author

The author spent his first five years eating, drinking, sleeping, getting toilet-trained, and learning how to draw with crayons. The next thirty years were spent in one or another school with the notable exception of a two-year stint in the U.S. Army. During that period, he managed to get one bachelor's degree, one master's, and two doctorates while avoiding any gainful employment. The next twenty-five years were spent having some sixty thousand patient office visits and performing north of ten thousand surgical procedures. He has written many articles that have appeared in such widely read magazines as *Biometrics* and *The Journal of the National Cancer Institute,* including the two page-turners "Misclassification in 2 by 2 Tables" and "A Statistical Model of the Natural History of Cervical Cancer." He co-authored a monograph on gynecological cancer with a Mr. Smith from Scotland. They were crushed when it didn't make it to the *New York Times* bestseller list.

Dr. Barron grossly underestimated the managed-care army forces. As late as 1995, he predicted that they would not occupy New York City until long after he had hung up his stethoscope for the last time and had like the old soldier of the famous barracks ballad just faded away. He was captured in 1996, and after resisting their brainwashing and assorted torture for some time, he appeared to be cooperating with the enemy. He cleverly escaped just before he was identified as a secret agent.

To this day, he considers himself lucky to have gotten away with his life. He was urged to write this book and agreed to do it, at some personal risk, in order to help you preserve yours.